Common Sense PREGNANCY

Common Sense
PREGNANCY

Navigating a Healthy
Pregnancy & Birth for
Mother & Baby

JEANNE FAULKNER, RN

TEN SPEED PRESS
Berkeley

Published in the United States by Ten Speed Press, an imprint of the Crown Publishing Group,
a division of Penguin Random House LLC, New York.
www.crownpublishing.com
www.tenspeed.com

Ten Speed Press and the Ten Speed Press colophon are registered trademarks of
Random House LLC.

Library of Congress Cataloging-in-Publication Data
Faulkner, Jeanne.
  Common sense pregnancy : navigating a healthy pregnancy and birth for mother and baby /
Jeanne Faulkner ; foreword by Christy Turlington and Erin Thornton.
    pages cm
  Summary: "JEANNE FAULKNER has worked in women's health for 30 years, first in doctor's
offices, free clinics, and classrooms and then as a registered nurse, specializing in obstetrics, labor
and delivery, and neonatal care. She began her career as a journalist in 2002 and currently writes
the weekly column Ask the Labor Nurse for FitPregnancy.com. She contributes articles about
health, medicine, food, parenting, travel, and lifestyle issues to such publications as Fit Pregnancy,
Pregnancy, Shape, Better Homes & Gardens, and the Huffington Post and Oregonian newspapers.
She's also the senior writer/editor for Every Mother Counts, a global maternal health advocacy
organization founded by Christy Turlington Burns — Provided by publisher.
  Includes bibliographical references and index.
  1. Pregnancy—Popular works. 2. Childbirth—Popular works. 3. Infants—Care—Popular works.
I. Title.
  RG525.F374 2015
  618.2—dc23
                        2015002870

Trade Paperback ISBN: 978-1-60774-675-1
eBook ISBN: 978-1-60774-676-8

Printed in the United States

Interior design by Chloe Rawlins
Cover design by Emma Campion
Cover illustration by Daphne Van Den Heuvel

10 9 8 7 6 5 4 3 2 1

First Edition

This book is dedicated to:

Phyllis, my mother and first love

Martha, Sedona, Peggy, and Kathy, my sisters

Jerome, Lauren, Camille, Lee, Olivia, and Lua, my family

And to all the parents and healthcare providers who are willing to change the way we think about, talk about, and experience pregnancy, birth, and parenting.

Contents

Foreword

BY CHRISTY TURLINGTON BURNS AND ERIN THORNTON

Becoming a mother is one of the most extraordinary things that can happen to a woman. It can and should be a beautiful, inspiring, empowering experience, but all too often it can also be confusing, scary, and overwhelming. Too many women experience the latter because many of them do not have access to the basic care and health care providers who can ensure a safe and happy experience. For some it's a lack of money and for some it's a matter of just physically getting there. For others, it's a matter of having the knowledge and support to have the best to pregnancy and childbirth experience possible.

Just as in most areas of life, knowledge is power and being aware of your options and having the ability to make choices is one way to ensure a healthy and positive birth experience. Having a reliable resource to help break down myth from fact is critical. Jeanne Faulkner has been the trusted resource behind the Every Mother Counts blog for years, translating the critical facts around maternal health into accessible, relatable content for mothers everywhere. When Erin needed support after the birth of her youngest daughter, Jeanne was on speed dial, cutting through the fluff and offering sound and steady advice when she needed it.

Now you can have Jeanne Faulkner on your speed dial, in the form of a book. *Common Sense Pregnancy* puts all of the most important information in one place and does so in the same direct, no-nonsense way that Jeanne would if she were on the other end of your phone. This book provides women with the information they truly need to understand pregnancy and childbirth, to know what to expect from their body, and to be equipped to make the right choices for them and their baby.

Every mother deserves a safe and healthy birth. Every mother deserves the opportunity to be in charge of her own birth experience. It may not always be pretty or fun, but the more that she knows and the more she can prepare herself and good make choices, the better an experience for everyone.

—Erin Thornton, executive director, and Christy Turlington Burns, founder of Every Mother Counts

Introduction

Information is the key to everything when you're pregnant. It's the key to your health, your baby's health, your relationship, your sex life, your birth plans, your mother-in-law, what underwear to buy, what fish you can eat—*everything*. Whether it's your first or tenth baby, you want to know all you can about this brand-new experience. After you talk to your doctor or midwife, mother, sister, and girlfriends, like most women you'll turn to books, magazines, and, more often than not, the modern mother of all resources—the Internet. That's where you'll find me writing FitPregnancy.com's *Ask the Labor Nurse* blog and global maternal health content for EveryMotherCounts.org. I'm a registered nurse and pregnancy/parenting/maternal health/advice blogger who's been in the women's and maternal health business for decades. Now I'm putting all my experience in one place: *Common Sense Pregnancy: A Common Sense Guide on How to Be Pregnant and Have a Baby*.

Making plans is an important part of pregnancy, but the best-laid plans can be conceived only with good information, lots of flexibility, and whopping doses of common sense. Even then, your plans and decisions aren't entirely up to you. There's a child involved, not to mention a partner, midwife, doctor, and family. It's complicated.

That's where I come in. I've spent decades working as a nurse in American hospitals, assisting with births from the most natural, low-intervention, and low-risk to the most high-risk and medically complicated, from water births to the ICU. I've been at the bedside for thousands of labors and deliveries—and I have four kids myself. I know that every pregnancy, birth, and child is unique, but also that there are only so many variations on what works and what doesn't, what's safe and what isn't. I've taken care of women of all ages, cultures, and demographics, and while my information is medically sound, not all of it is what you'll hear from your doctor. Because I've worked so long "on the inside," I can tell you what to really expect during pregnancy and delivery. You may be surprised to learn that most of it is good news.

I've also spent years immersed in the global maternal health world as an advocate for the international humanitarian organization CARE and as senior writer and editor for a global maternal health advocacy organization. And from this depth of experience, I've learned a few things about what we do right here in the United States, what needs improvement, and how important common sense is during pregnancy, birth, and parenting.

The traditional U.S. medical model for maternal health care is anchored in fear and treats pregnancy and childbirth as a disease. It is complication-based and mired in legally defendable health care policies and insurance requirements that can seem scary as hell. For example, your doctor may tell you about your increased risks for certain complications and design your prenatal care and birth around those risks. Most mothers never develop most complications; nevertheless, routine prenatal and delivery care still revolve around risks. Doctors recommend routine interventions to forestall those (for most women, nonexistent) risks, but they don't always inform patients that unnecessary medical interventions have risks, too.

Some medical interventions are excellent and lead to kinder, gentler, and safer births, but in this day and age of extreme and polarizing opinions on pregnancy, childbirth, and parenting, that's not how they're presented in many media outlets.

It's time to dial down the drama in the American birth industry and dial up a heavy dose of common sense. With C-sections performed in a third of our births, women fighting for their rights to deliver safely, and doctors so stressed out and exhausted they're abandoning obstetrics in droves, it's time to make some changes. Real change places maternal health practices back in the land of evidence-based standards of care.

Real change creates policies and practices that empower and support women *and* health care providers. It takes the fear out of being pregnant, because most pregnancies are safe when we have access to common sense information.

Common Sense Pregnancy is similar to the e-conversation I have with my online readers—part Q&A, part memoir, and part straight-up medical information. It's informed by my personal and professional experience, and it provides a multifaceted peek at one of the most common experiences known to womankind.

You can read this book one piece at a time, or settle in and read several sections. Together, let's dial up the common sense as you prepare for pregnancy, birth, and parenthood.

CHAPTER 1

When You First Get Pregnant

Now that you're honest-to-goodness pregnant, let's get down to business and answer some of the questions every pregnant woman has.

In this book, we're going to cover everything from figuring out how to adapt your daily life to pregnancy to how to decide on genetic testing to everything you need to know about ultrasounds. Then we'll dig into some of the less commonly asked questions, like: how about sex? And what if I did drugs? Being pregnant is complicated, but don't worry—you've got this. Let's get it all straightened out.

What to do when you find out you're pregnant

You've taken the test and it came out positive. It's official. You're pregnant. Now what?

At first? Do nothing. Absorb this moment. It's literally the most life-changing moment of your life. If there were ever a moment to BE HERE NOW, this is it. Breathe in, breathe out. Be still.

What if the news of your pregnancy isn't met with immediate happiness? Well, then, you have some big adjustments to make. If you're feeling undercurrents of uncertainty, know that you're among friends. Every woman feels at least a few uncomfortable feelings, no matter how welcome the news. If your pregnancy is occurring at an inopportune time in your life, you'll just feel these a little more. My advice? Right now, do nothing. Sit still. Absorb this moment. Be here now. Repeat as often as necessary until you feel less distressed, weird, or scared.

Don't feel rushed to do anything other than to take really good care of yourself. Treat yourself gently. Baby yourself, as you will your newborn—because right now, you are your own baby. You are at the beginning of the biggest change in your life, and your ability to embrace this change depends entirely on the level of compassion you give yourself. If you feel like you're walking in a fog—you are, so embrace it.

If you're partnered or married, your partner is going to need gentle treatment and compassion, too, because he or she is also going through a huge change. Be kind to each other. This is how you'll set the tone for the rest of your life as parents. Pretty soon things will start changing fast, but for this moment, just sit with the news that you are pregnant. That's enough for now.

How to have a well pregnancy instead of a fear-based pregnancy

You know those optical illusions you stare and stare at, seeing only one thing? What do you see, a vase or two faces? The longer you focus, the more your mind commits to seeing only one image. It isn't until you make a subtle shift that suddenly you see a second image, too. It was there all along, right in front of your eyes, but until you looked at it differently, you couldn't see anything else.

That's kind of what happens to a lot of women during pregnancy. Some women see pregnancy as completely normal and healthy with no potential for complications. Others see pregnancy as freaky and weird, risky and dangerous. Still others see both sides—the normalcy and the risk—and make a choice as to which image to focus on.

That's also kind of what happens with our two main medical models for receiving health care during pregnancy. There's the midwifery model of care, which focuses on pregnancy as a normal physiologic process, and there's the obstetric model, which focuses on the potential risks associated with pregnancy. Both models are important, and each works best when it's integrated with the other and practiced appropriately. When either model insists we see pregnancy through only that lens, we tend to develop blind spots.

Most pregnancies and births progress with no complications whatsoever. Every pregnancy, however, holds an element of risk. The difference between a well pregnancy and a fear-based pregnancy is which part you focus on—the mostly normal healthy parts or the potentially risky parts. If you focus primarily on being healthy, staying well, and supporting your body to do a bang-up job at growing your baby, chances are very good you'll enjoy a well pregnancy and childbirth and welcome a healthy baby. That's what a well pregnancy looks like. If you focus primarily on potential complications, you may support those fears with medical care that shares that focus. That's what a fear-based pregnancy looks like.

Some women come to pregnancy with a medical history and health conditions that require more focus on the potential for developing complications. Some women enter pregnancy 100-percent healthy, then develop complications along the way. This subset of women with complicated pregnancies makes up approximately 15 percent of all the pregnant mamas out there. Their health depends on acknowledging that their body needs more support to stay well and deliver a healthy baby. That's what a well pregnancy looks like for women with complicated medical histories. Thank goodness high-quality obstetric care is available to shepherd these women and their babies safely through to motherhood.

Most women (about 85 percent), however, are just fine and really don't need all the bells and whistles that come with high-risk obstetric care. The problem is, the obstetric model is the most common, easily accessible, widely accepted model of care, used by about 86 percent of mothers. The other 14 percent use non-OB providers like midwives and family practice doctors. Because obstetricians are educated, trained, and skilled at dealing with medical complications in pregnancy, it's only natural that most focus on the potential risks. Their model of care is designed to rule out and ward off complications by doing extra tests and treatments. Add to that the heavy weight of medical malpractice insurance—which to a large extent dictates how they practice, to make sure they don't make any mistakes—and there you have it: they see a vase instead of the face, even though they know the face is right there.

In many countries with really excellent maternal health outcomes, all the normal, healthy women see midwives for prenatal and childbirth care. If a problem develops (and midwives are trained to recognize problems), they transfer care to an obstetrician. It's a model of care that makes a lot of sense.

Whenever possible, I think most women in the United States should see midwives during pregnancy and delivery, because these experts are the naturals at recognizing pregnancy as a normal physiologic event, not a medical crisis to be managed. That paradigm shift isn't going to happen overnight, though. The key to having a well pregnancy for women accessing traditional obstetric care is to insist on a well-pregnancy focus over a risk-based focus. It also requires that more women let go of their fears and focus on their role: being well.

How can you dial down the fear in your pregnancy? By flipping your focus from illness to wellness, and by going with the most appropriate type of health care for you. For most women, there's just not that much to worry about. Yes, there are risks for complications, but they're relatively small, and most women won't develop them. We'll talk a lot about that in subsequent sections, but for every mother, whether you have medical complications or you're 100-percent healthy, having a well pregnancy requires that you:

- Be an active participant in your health by doing everything you can to be healthy.

- Be an active participant in your health care by being picky about which interventions you consent to and which ones are simply not necessary.

- Go with the lowest intervention level that's appropriate for you, not the rule-everything-out, high-risk model that's become one-size-fits-all for women.

Don't let fear terrorize your pregnancy. Focus on what's real: Unless you have some real honest-to-goodness health problems, you're most likely going to have a healthy pregnancy. As long as you're safe, wellnourished, taking care of yourself, and not living in danger, then your odds for having a perfectly normal pregnancy and childbirth are excellent. In fact, you're at increased risk for normalcy and health. How do you like those odds?

Is your pregnancy no-risk, low-risk, moderate-risk, or high-risk?

When you're reading up on prenatal health care options and interventions, you'll see the terms "low-risk" and "high-risk," as in, "She had a high-risk pregnancy and needed an emergency C-section," or "She was a low-risk patient, so we were surprised when she developed complications." What exactly do risk levels mean?

First off, let's get one category off the table. No pregnancy is ever considered *no-risk*. Every pregnancy carries risk, but risk doesn't necessarily mean harm, injury, illness, or death. The word *risk* has two meanings in a medical setting.

1: The *possibility* of loss or injury to a patient.

2: The *possibility* that a patient will sue a provider or cause an insurance company to pay for damages incurred.

In both cases, the definition hinges on one word: possibility. Possibility does not mean guarantee. It means something *might* happen, but in all likelihood it won't. Every pregnancy has the possibility of injury or death, and every pregnancy could end in a lawsuit if something bad happens to mother or baby, regardless of whether the provider is at fault. With every single pregnancy there's the possibility that something could go wrong, but I'll say it again: in the vast majority of cases, everything turns out just fine.

How do you know if you're low-risk, moderate-risk, or high-risk? We start with a list of high-risk factors and conditions. If nothing on this list applies to you, you're low-risk.

You're *potentially* high-risk if:

- You're older than thirty-five or younger than fifteen
- You have high blood pressure or a history of preeclampsia or eclampsia

  or

- Kidney problems
- Autoimmune disorders
- Diabetes
- Cancer
- Asthma (uncontrolled)
- Seizure disorder
- Obesity or extreme underweight
- More than one fetus
- History of gestational diabetes
- History of premature labor or premature baby
- History of baby with birth defects or health complications
- Any other serious or chronic health condition

Some of those problems are a bigger deal than others. You could have conditions on this list and be considered to be in only a moderate-risk category. For example, well-controlled asthma or a history of cancer that's cured doesn't automatically make you high-risk. You could also start out as a low-risk patient, then develop high-risk issues during pregnancy, like placental complications, intrauterine growth retardation, premature rupture of membranes, Rh incompatibility, infections, and others. That's why high-quality prenatal care is essential to all mothers.

How many women have low-risk pregnancies? According to Healthy People 2020, a U.S. Department of Health and Human Services resource organization, 85 percent, or 3.5 million, of the American women who have babies each year are considered to have low-risk pregnancies. They have good reason to expect an uncomplicated birth and a healthy newborn.

Why are risk levels important?

Risk factors and risk levels drive many of the standards of care that determine how women are treated as patients during pregnancy. Because the American health care system is based on private or public insurance every woman is considered a potential risk. Her prenatal care will be directed toward lowering the odds she'll incur harm and/or sue her doctor. Not every health care provider views patients that way, but many do, which is why they order tons of tests to rule out potential risks, just in case—whether or not their patient really needs those tests and whether or not it will improve her health. Most doctors and many midwives take a "let's just not take any chances" attitude.

Doctors, some midwives, and hospitals that intervene by doing tests, treatments, and procedures are motivated partly to provide good care, partly to generate revenue, but also partly to ensure that if they wind up in court they can prove they did everything possible for their patient. Obstetricians who are too intent on finding or ruling out complications on healthy women may intervene medically when it's not really necessary. Unfortunately, doing everything in the medical manual isn't safe either and sometimes increases risk factors for loss and injury. We've learned in recent years that interventions done unnecessarily (for instance, induction of labor for nonmedical reasons) often lead to more interventions (like the C-section that results after that induction fails to progress, and the subsequent C-sections that the mother will mostly likely undergo with future pregnancies). That's a major reason why we're seeing increased maternal and newborn injuries and deaths in the United States resulting in large part from out-of-control C-section rates.

Are doctors doing extra interventions because they're more profitable? Some may be, no doubt, but most probably aren't. Most are just practicing medicine the way they've been trained, the way their hospitals mandate, and the way they're required to by their malpractice insurers in order to be medically defensible in court.

What's the solution to the increasingly risk-driven birth industry? We're figuring that out on a case-by-case basis, but for now, it all has to do with how healthy a particular woman is before she becomes pregnant. Low-risk women have more options than high-risk women in terms of the kind of provider, birth style, and setting they can use. A truly healthy woman can potentially deliver safely at home with a skilled midwife if she wants to, or at a birth center, or in a hospital—essentially, wherever she chooses. High-risk patients' options, on the other hand, are limited to hospitals because they need specialists like obstetricians, perinatologists, and maternal-fetal medicine experts.

Even women who are diagnosed as high risk can have absolutely normal, healthy pregnancies and births. In fact, given the opportunity, most do. It's an amazing time in medical history for pregnant women. Even as recently as thirty or forty years ago, many high-risk women were advised to not get pregnant. Nowadays, many are encouraged to "go for it" because we have the treatments and technologies to make even high-risk pregnancies relatively safe.

On the other end of the spectrum, even the lowest-risk women can develop unforeseen complications and wind up in the intensive care unit or worse. Pregnancy and childbirth are unpredictable like that. The chances that you're in that entirely normal 85 percent, however, are darn good, which raises the question: Why are so many women treated like high-risk patients when they're actually in that low-risk category? Because the way we manage health care and obstetrics here in the United States is seriously messed up. The good news is, experts are realizing that the way we've been operating lately is causing needless harm, and things have to change.

Part of that change requires that women do all they can to lower their risks, opt for care providers who respect that pregnancy and birth are usually normal, and demand a better model of care. It's a two-way street—both women and health care providers have to do better.

How soon do you need to see a midwife or doctor?

A woman I know (I'll call her Dionne) recently announced her first pregnancy about twenty minutes after she missed her period. She's super excited and more than a little nervous. When she called her doctor's office to make her first prenatal appointment, she was annoyed and, frankly, frightened because her doctor said he'd see her when she was eight weeks pregnant. That's six weeks away! What the heck is Dionne supposed to do now?

Christina scheduled her first prenatal appointment for twelve weeks. She'd seen her midwife recently for a well-woman exam and knew she was perfectly healthy. She was already taking vitamins, didn't want a bunch of testing, and knew if she needed anything, her midwife was just a phone call away.

Adele called her midwife to let her know her pregnancy test was positive, and she was whisked into the first available appointment, just a few days later. Adele is as healthy as can be, but she had an early miscarriage last year, which left her feeling fragile. Her midwife wanted to start supporting her ASAP.

And then there's Lisa. She's thirty-eight and has been undergoing infertility treatments for over a year. This is the first time the pregnancy test has come out positive. She's just a little overweight, her blood pressure is just a little higher than normal, and in her quest to get pregnant she's been seeing doctors for what feels like forever. As soon as she and her doctors knew this round of treatments had succeeded, they shifted gears and started calling her appointments *prenatal care*.

As you see from these four stories, the answer to the question "How soon do you need to see a midwife or doctor?" is, "It depends." If you're healthy, like Dionne and Christina, and you've never had any previous pregnancy complications like the ones Adele and Lisa have, then you don't really *need* to see a doctor or midwife during the first month or two of pregnancy.

Not much that your health care provider does during the earliest weeks of pregnancy will make much difference to your health or your baby's health. It's too early to see much on ultrasound (which at this point would be done mostly for fun or to confirm you're really, truly pregnant) and too early for first trimester screening exams. You don't really need a pelvic exam or Pap smear (the routine test for cervical cancer). In fact, some women think that having a Pap done during the first trimester may lead to miscarriage. It won't. Pap smears aren't invasive enough to cause miscarriage. They can, however, irritate a particularly sensitive cervix, and they can cause light spotting, which makes newly pregnant women nervous. That's partly why some doctors and midwives prefer to wait until late in the first trimester before they see patients.

That's why Dionne's doctor said, "Pick up some prenatal vitamins at the store. I'll see you in six weeks." That's plenty soon enough to do blood tests and a physical exam, and eight weeks is about the soonest anyone can hear a teeny tiny heartbeat.

Call your doctor (or midwife, if you already have one) fairly soon after you know you're pregnant, and they'll let you know how soon you need to be seen. If you haven't chosen a provider yet and want to shop around, call a few docs and/or midwives and schedule some meet-and-greets before you commit to a specific provider. Then go with the provider who's most convenient and most aligned with your health care goals and who makes you feel most cared for. (For more on choosing a health care provider, see page 25.)

But what if problems develop in the first few weeks, like nausea or extreme fatigue or a little bit of spotting? Just because you don't have an appointment scheduled in the immediate future doesn't mean you can't call your provider and ask for support. If you're feeling so sick you're barfing up your socks, your doctor might say, "Let's see you this afternoon." Severe morning sickness—a rare form called hyperemesis gravidarum—can be so debilitating you may need medication or even IV hydration (more on this later). If you're so tired you can't get out of bed, your provider might say, "Welcome to the club, now go take a nap," but she might also say, "Come on in tomorrow and let's make sure everything's OK." There might not be anything in particular from a medical standpoint your provider can do to make you feel any better, but she can provide sympathy, compassion, and reassurance, which can be more valuable than almost anything else.

If you're spotting a little, your doctor might say, "Wait and see." Early spotting during the first trimester does not necessarily indicate a problem. About 20 to 30 percent of pregnant women have light spotting during the first trimester, and about half of those "spotters" miscarry.[1] The half who don't miscarry are experiencing either implantation bleeding (when the fetus imbeds into the uterine lining), cervical irritation (caused by hormones and fragile blood vessels in the cervix), or discharge of old menstrual blood, and the spotting stops without treatment. In other words, for them it's a normal part of pregnancy—though admittedly annoying and a bit frightening. (For more about spotting and its causes, see page 55.)

If the spotting is the precursor to an early miscarriage, there's little or nothing your doctor or midwife can do to prevent it. If the spotting stops—excellent! Chances are good you'll be fine. If it doesn't stop or it gets heavier, call your midwife or doctor. If you're having a miscarriage, your provider will determine what kind of care you need—compassionate handholding while the miscarriage takes place on its own, or a medical procedure called dilation and curettage (D&C) to empty your uterus.

I hate to end on a sad note, so let's do my favorite thing. Let's flip the statistics. While 15 to 20 percent of women will experience a miscarriage, most occur before a woman even knows she's pregnant. We rarely know what causes a miscarriage, though prevailing wisdom says it's Mother Nature's way of ending a pregnancy that was destined for problems, like genetic anomalies. The good news is that most women who have early miscarriages go on to eventually have entirely normal, healthy pregnancies in the future. An even more positive take: 80 to 85 percent of all pregnancies *do not* miscarry.

When it comes right down to it, the most important part of good prenatal care is reassurance that everything is OK. While the earliest weeks of pregnancy may be a time when you need that reassurance more than ever, it's not a time that most women need much medical care. Turn to your mother, sister, grandmother, aunt, girlfriend, or some other trusted, loved, experienced woman. Turn to your partner. Most important, turn to yourself and know that your body has its own wisdom. Take care of yourself physically, mentally, and emotionally and the odds are in your favor that you and your baby will be fine.

Who should you tell that you're pregnant, and when?

Who is the first person you want to tell after the pee stick turns positive? For most of you, it's going to be your partner. If you're happy as heck that you're pregnant, you'll want to share it with the person who helped you get that way. If your feelings are mixed (let's face it—finding out you're pregnant can feel overwhelming and the news can bring as much anxiety as joy, for any number of reasons) all the more reason to start gathering your tribe around you. Whoever it is, however you feel, tell someone right away. You need, want, deserve support. This is news that's so big it needs to be shared.

Once you've told your most significant insider your big news, sit back and let it soak in. There's no prescribed time period you have to wait, but this news will be yours and your partner's alone for only a short time. Once word gets out, it will spread, and that's when your pregnancy and baby start belonging to others. It will be your mother's grandchild you're carrying, your brother's niece or nephew, your best friend's "first baby." Your coworkers' office baby. It's not just your pregnancy anymore, just as this won't be just your child. As soon as you spill the beans, your child will be part of your family, a member of your community.

Who you tell next is up for debate. Personally, I think there's a hierarchy or order of notification that should be honored. If your partner is first, your parents should be second, your partner's parents third, then your siblings and best friends. After that—it's a free-for-all. If the rest of your universe hasn't already heard the news, have fun telling them whenever, wherever you want.

Before any of you say, "I don't want my mom to know right away": that's fine. Believe me, this order of notification isn't carved in stone. What I want you to get is this: the order in which you tell people may carry major relationship consequences. Give yourself time to think it through.

A friend of mine recently discovered she was unexpectedly pregnant. She wasn't unhappy about it, but she was caught by surprise. Her husband was delighted, and after a minor period of adjustment, she was too. When she told me her news, she said, "I'm not supposed to tell anyone until I'm past the first trimester, right?"

I answered, "Where'd you get that idea? Is there a Pregnancy Rule Book I'm unaware of?"

"Well," she said, "if anything happens [code-speak for miscarriage] and everyone already knows I'm pregnant, well then . . . I mean . . . it's better if I don't have to tell everyone that news. Right?"

My answer surprised her. "Honey, you get to tell anyone you want, as soon as you want. If 'something happens,' you'll need some friends and family to help you through the grief. Maybe you're not ready to share the news with your entire clan, but there are no rules that mandate you have to keep your pregnancy secret until you've reached a safe period."

It's weird that in our society we think women shouldn't share their pregnancy because they might miscarry—as if they're going to jinx it by telling. It's even weirder that women who miscarry are expected to suffer in silence—that it's supposed to be better if no one knows. It's as if we don't want to trouble anyone with our anxiety that something might happen to our fragile pregnancy or burden them with our sadness if something does happen. But is it better for women to feel alone and unsupported through these huge emotional issues? There *are* some good reasons to keep a lid on who you tell and how soon, but fear of miscarriage shouldn't be one of them.

What are those good reasons? As I've said, one of the best reasons to delay spreading the news is to keep your experience all to yourself for a while. But other reasons include:

- You don't want to deal with other peoples' reactions.

- You're embarrassed or afraid you'll be judged or teased ("What? Pregnant again?") and you're feeling fragile.

- You don't want your employers to know until you've figured out a motherhood-work strategy.

- You're in a bad relationship and don't want your exit strategy complicated by your partner's reaction.

How do you tell people? There's a growing trend to make it a really big deal. I've heard about flash mobs of choreographed dancers turning the news into a big Broadway number. Some women get fortune cookies delivered with their take-out Chinese food with the message "I'm pregnant" baked inside. Some women drop the pregnancy test into a plastic bag and hide it in their husband's gym bag or briefcase. There are a million ways to go big on this news that can be a lot of fun. Go for it if that's your style, but let's be careful that the telling doesn't upstage the news itself. Seriously, it's already exciting that you're pregnant and bringing a brand-new human into your life. It's a baby. That's big enough.

How soon will you look pregnant instead of just fluffy?

Pregnant bellies go through four phases:

1. Your stomach looks just like it did prepregnancy.
2. You look like you've gained weight, but don't necessarily look pregnant.
3. There's no doubt about it—you look pregnant.
4. You look like you're ready to pop.

What's the best phase? Most women pick phase three, when they're past the "I've gained weight" stage and full on into the "I look pregnant" stage. There's no set schedule as to when you'll reach this stage. First-time mothers tend to *show* (the traditional term for "she looks pregnant") later than mothers who've been pregnant before. Overweight women often show later too, and very thin women tend to show a bit earlier. Women with super strong abdominal muscles might get well into their second trimester before anyone notices their tummy. Women with twins or triplets? Way earlier than mothers of single babies.

As a general guideline, most first-time mothers of single babies start feeling like their pants are too tight between 10 and 12 weeks. It's not that their baby is all that big, but the uterus is growing to accommodate a placenta, amniotic fluid, and extra blood volume. Constipation is also very common during pregnancy and, when combined with gas and bloating, might make your stomach look fuller. Your skin may feel extra sensitive too, which motivates many women to buy softer, stretchier pants, even if they don't really need maternity jeans yet. By 14 weeks, most women need to either unbutton their waistband, go shopping in the maternity department, or borrow their partner's sweatpants.

You can get away with wearing your own clothes longer if you unbutton/unzip and fasten your pants with a rubber band or a loop of elastic. Wear longer shirts (or not, if you want to show off your belly) and you can go quite a ways into your pregnancy without having to shop. The benefit of wearing maternity duds is, they're cut in a way that emphasizes your baby bump and takes some of the guesswork out of the "is she or isn't she?" question.

By the time they're at 20 weeks, most women look undeniably pregnant. If you're still not showing, don't worry that it means anything's wrong. Your midwife or doctor will be checking you out at your prenatal visits to make sure your baby is growing normally.

If phase one feels like you're keeping a secret (no one can tell you're pregnant), then phase two feels like you're posing a question (is she pregnant?). Phase three provides the answer (yep, she's pregnant). Phase four is the one that causes women the most trouble, because some women's bellies get so big, they look like labor must be imminent even weeks to months before their due date. I carried right out front; with each of my pregnancies, at about seven months people started telling me with absolute certainty that either I was having twins or I was going to deliver any day. Let it be a testament to my excellent character and upbringing that I never punched one single person in the mouth when they said it; not even that one lady who told me that I obviously didn't know my due date because she could always tell when a woman was about to go into labor.

What does your due date really mean?

Finding out your due date is kind of like circling a date for magic to happen. It's a bit like choosing your wedding date, for all the planning, excitement, and anticipation that goes into it. It's also like graduation, because—particularly if it's your first child—you'll be completing one phase of your life and entering into an entirely new one. But unlike your wedding or graduation dates, a due date *is not* an exact day when you'll deliver your baby. It's just an estimate of more or less when your baby might be born. If that sounds unspecific and tentative, then great—you're getting my drift.

Your due date (aka estimated date of confinement, or EDC) is just a best-guess estimate based on the average length of a normal pregnancy. It's calculated as 280 days, or 40 weeks, or 9 months and 7 days after the first day of your last menstrual period (LMP). The easy way to calculate it, *if* you know when your last period started, is to go back three months and add seven days and voilà—your due date.

But here's the kicker—only about 5 percent of women go into labor on their due date. The other 95 percent deliver a few days or even weeks before or after, and for most, that's entirely normal.

What if you don't know the first date of your LMP? Then your doctor will pick a due date based on an ultrasound. The earlier the ultrasound is done, the more accurate the due date, though those based on first-trimester ultrasounds may be off by as much as a week. Estimates based on ultrasounds done in the second or third trimester are notoriously inaccurate; they can be off by as much as two weeks before or after when the baby is actually due to deliver spontaneously without medical intervention.

Most women get pregnant approximately two weeks after their last period started, and the two weeks before conception are counted as part of the length of pregnancy. That's because unless your baby is conceived under very special circumstances (in vitro fertilization, for example) it's difficult to know exactly when you got pregnant. You'd have to calculate the speed at which sperm travels and the proximity of the egg released at ovulation, and frankly, that's just too much algebra and technology for most babies. Therefore, your due date is based on a 40-week pregnancy, which gives everybody a bit of wiggle room.

It is not, however, an ironclad commitment that you will absolutely have your baby on that date. This is important, because when your due date is coming close or has come and gone, you and your provider may be so eager to get that baby delivered that you start messing with Mother Nature's day-planner. Your doctor may start hinting at an induction before your due date's even arrived or might say he won't "let you" go past your due date. Your mother might pester you to walk for miles or eat spicy food to get things started. Your best friend might tell you to have lots of sex to start contractions. People tend to treat due dates like deadlines, and if you don't deliver on time, well then, something must be wrong.

There's even more pressure to get the show on the road if you go past your due date. Statistically speaking, about 31.5 percent of women deliver sometime between their 40th week (due date) and their 41st, and about 16 percent deliver between 41 and 42 weeks.[2] That is, if the pregnancy is left to finish on its own terms and labor is not induced or the baby delivered by C-section. Excluding the women who deliver prematurely (about 12.3 percent of births), everybody else starts labor within a few days of their due date.

There's a huge shift happening in the medical community to quit putting so much emphasis on delivering by the due date. There's a lot of finish work to be completed before a baby is ready to leave the womb and live life independently from its mother. We got into a bad habit during the 1980s and 1990s of routinely short-changing babies by scheduling unnecessary inductions, and we ended up delivering a lot of premature babies. Midwives have been saying, "Leave mothers alone" for decades, but the American Congress of Obstetricians and Gynecologists only recently got on board with the idea that maybe mothers and babies know best (most of the time, anyway) about when baby should be born. In fact, they recently revamped their guidelines about what they consider term or due:[3]

RECOMMENDED CLASSIFICATION OF DELIVERIES FROM 37 WEEKS OF GESTATION

· Early term: 37 0/7 weeks through 38 6/7 weeks
· Full term: 39 0/7 weeks through 40 6/7 weeks
· Late term: 41 0/7 weeks through 41 6/7 weeks
· Post-term: 42 0/7 weeks and beyond

According to this, you're not overdue (post-term) until two weeks past your due date.[4] That's how iffy a due date is. You can't count on it. You can only hope for it. And even then, in most cases, it's best to assume your body knows better than your calendar when to deliver.

How much stuff do you need?

When you visit a baby store for the first time as a soon-to-be parent, expect to have a panic attack. Sure, you've been to these stores before. You've shopped for baby shower presents; no big deal, right? Wrong. Shopping for one little gift is nothing compared to shopping in preparation for your baby's life. The list of essential products, furniture, clothes, and gear you're expected to purchase is so daunting and huge that unless you have a personal shopper and a never-ending bank account, you're going to freak out. Here's my best piece of advice on that—relax! You don't actually need most of that stuff.

Think back to every generation raised before about a hundred years ago (that is, before commercial manufacturing, technology, and consumerism kicked into high gear). What did those parents need to survive babyhood? Somewhere for baby to sleep (a bottom drawer of the dresser worked just fine), a couple dozen cloth diapers, some blankets and clothes, and maybe a toy. That's it. These babies survived childhood well enough that they created Greco-Roman architecture, the Industrial Revolution, cars, and penicillin; they survived the Great Depression, developed rock 'n' roll—you get my point. It wasn't the *stuff* parents had when their babies were little that created their children's platform for growth. It was something else entirely.

Somewhere along the line, we became the child-centered, consumer-driven society we are today, and marketers discovered that parents will buy all kinds of crap thinking they *need* it to raise a superior child. Sure, some of those products are genius—baby wipes, comfortable baby carriers, Velcro diaper covers, disposable diapers, car seats, strollers. But an awful lot of it is absolutely unnecessary and I think creates competition, distraction, and insecurity among parents. Do you need a thousand-dollar stroller to help your baby go places in the world? Nope.

A custom-made breastfeeding pillow to get the best latch? Nope. How about a top o' the line crib that converts into a toddler bed to cultivate good sleep habits? Nope. Toys that stimulate your baby's brain so he'll get into Harvard? Nope. Ergonomically designed silverware so your baby will develop manners, culinary discernment, and a refined palate? Nope, nope, nope.

Here's what you need to get started:

- Somewhere for your baby to sleep. A basket, cosleeper, bassinet, crib—whatever works. Just make sure it's safe. Check out safety guidelines and recommendations in baby-centered magazines and shopping guides and maybe *Consumer Reports*.

- Something to keep her warm. Buy enough blankets and clothes to keep her warm, dry, and clean for three days without doing laundry. Don't overdress or put too much stuff in her bed.

- Something to keep him safe in the car. Get the newest car seat you can afford, but don't spend too much. They outgrow them quickly.

- Something to carry baby in. A stroller, a carrier, a sling—whatever's easy on your back and lets you get from place to place while keeping your hands relatively free.

- Something to keep her butt dry. Cloth, disposable, organic, and generic diapers all have their own environmental and economic advantages. You'll have to work that out on your own. If you go for cloth, you'll also need safety pins and plastic pants or Velcro-fastened covers. Stock up on enough to get you through three days or more without doing laundry.

- Some way to feed him. If you're breastfeeding, you have almost everything you need right on your chest. You'll also need a few nursing bras and pads to accommodate your bigger, leakier breasts. If someone gives you a breastfeeding pillow—sweet! If not, use ordinary pillows and folded blankets to create your own. You may need some nipple cream, a breast pump, and a few other odds and ends to store your milk, but you may not. Wait and see. And see chapter 16 on how to feed your baby.

- If you're bottlefeeding, you'll need bottles, nipples, formula, and bottle cleaners. Go for bottles that are BPA-free, and buy enough to get through a day without washing dishes.

There—you're done. Your shopping list will undoubtedly be less austere than this one, and that's perfectly OK. A lot of the stuff you'll see in the baby store is fun, helpful, cute, and convenient, and if you can afford it or someone gives it to you, what the heck—go for it. Don't confuse the fun with thinking you *need* it. You don't. Don't go thinking you'll be a better parent if you have more stuff. You won't. Don't assume newer is better. It probably isn't. Use hand-me-downs whenever possible; check out the baby consignment shops and thrift stores. Share your stuff with your friends when you're done with it.

Simplify and save your money for the things your child really needs. They'll let you know what those things are as they grow. Splurge on activities over stuff, because the toys will break, but the memories you create together as a family will be there for a lifetime. And don't go crazy with the "smart toys," because it doesn't really matter whether or not you buy the latest electronic gadget. Babies and small children are happy with very little. On a final note, save your money for what really matters, because if you're hoping your baby is going to college someday, it is ridiculously expensive.

CHAPTER 2

Choosing Your Care

We talked a little in chapter 1 about how obstetric and midwifery models of care differ and about how other countries with top-notch maternal health outcomes use midwives more often than obstetricians. We also talked about why some women need more advanced obstetric care than others. Here in chapter 2, we'll cover the differences between varying types of maternal care providers, how to pick the best care provider for you, how to create a labor support team, and where to deliver your baby. This is where you start taking the reins of your prenatal care.

How to pick your health care provider

American women have lots of options when choosing a health care provider to see during pregnancy—a midwife, naturopath, family practice doctor, or obstetrician. Your choice depends on your insurance provider (if you have one), where you live, your health, and your preferred type of health care.

You have fewer choices, however, when it comes to who will be present when you deliver. It used to be that whoever provided your prenatal care was also the one who delivered the baby. Now women often see one provider (or more) during their pregnancy and whoever is on call (probably a different doctor/midwife in their provider's practice) during labor and birth. Some hospitals currently employ laborists (aka hospitalists)—obstetricians who work in the maternity unit to care for women in labor and delivery. You may or may not have ever met this doctor before he or she shows up to deliver your baby. That means that unless you choose a provider who guarantees he or she will be there when you deliver, you're in for luck-of-the-draw. Some women are perfectly fine with that, but others find the uncertainty a bit unsettling. I get that, but I wouldn't worry too much. It's part of a laborist's and on-call doctor's job to ease your transition from seeing her as a stranger to trusting that you and your baby are in good hands with her. If there's time after you arrive at the hospital in labor and before you deliver your baby, tell your provider about your birth plans, then keep calm and carry on.

The Affordable Care Act of 2010 mandates that virtually all U.S. insurance plans cover prenatal care, delivery services, and hospital stay. Your plan may let you choose any midwife or doctor you want, or you may have to choose from a preauthorized list of providers. If you aren't insured, check with your county health department to see if you're eligible for state-sponsored insurance, or shop around for the most affordable prenatal care options and payment plans.

Your choice of provider will greatly depend on your health. Choose a provider who specializes in taking care of women in your risk category. If you're healthy and at low risk for complications, a midwife may be your perfect choice. If you have health problems that might affect your pregnancy, an obstetrician and possibly other specialists may be a better option.

Your preferred *type of health care* refers to whether you prefer traditional or alternative care. If you usually see a naturopath, chiropractor, or acupuncturist, you may feel most comfortable seeing a midwife for prenatal care. If you're used to seeing an internist or other medical specialist for routine health care, you may feel more comfortable seeing a doctor. But keep an open mind: you may find midwifery care a refreshing change of style. After you've made your first choice—doctor or a midwife—your next choice is what *type* of doctor or midwife. There are lots of options to choose from.

Many doctors of naturopathy, family practice doctors, doctors of osteopathy, and medical doctors practice obstetrics.

Naturopaths (NDs) are doctors of naturopathic medicine. They study all the same sciences as medical doctors, plus holistic and nontoxic therapies, nutrition, acupuncture, homeopathy, and psychology.

Some NDs also complete an additional two years of training in midwifery. NDs can't deliver babies in hospitals, but some deliver in homes and birth centers.

Doctors of osteopathy (DOs) have all the same medical privileges as medical doctors (MDs) and practice the full scope of Western medicine and the same range of specialties as MDs. DOs take a slightly different educational pathway, but they can prescribe drugs, perform surgeries, and practice in all the same hospitals and locations as MDs in the United States. Many specialize in obstetrics.

Medical doctors (MDs) are the practitioners whom people traditionally think of as *doctors*. **Family practice doctors** are MDs or DOs who treat patients of all ages. Some provide prenatal care to low- to moderate-risk patients and deliver babies. They also provide pediatric care to newborns. They aren't obstetricians, so if problems arise, they'll consult with one.

Obstetricians (OBs) are either MDs or DOs who specialize in prenatal care, labor, birth, high-risk pregnancy, and surgery. Most prenatal patients in the United States see OBs. That's the model of care we've become accustomed to over many decades. Just because a specific doctor is a specialist in high-risk patients doesn't necessarily mean she will view all her patients as potentially high-risk.

When choosing a specific doctor, find out what their C-section rate is and what interventions they prefer. I've worked with OBs you'd swear were actually midwives because of their hands-on, low-intervention approach and high rates of vaginal birth. I've also worked with OBs who'd make every birth a C-section if that were possible. It's the doctor, not the license, that makes the difference.

Midwives have different licensures, levels of experience, and areas of expertise. There are certified nurse midwives, certified professional midwives, direct entry midwives, and lay midwives.

- **Certified nurse-midwives (CNMs)** are registered nurses who have graduated from an accredited nurse-midwifery education program and passed a national certification examination. CNMs practice legally in hospitals, birth centers, and private homes in all fifty states.

- **Certified midwives (CMs)** come from health backgrounds other than nursing. They graduate from accredited midwifery education programs, take the same national certification examination as CNMs, and can practice legally in many states. The difference between CMs and CNMs is the nursing component, which doesn't necessarily make a difference to their practice.

- **Certified professional midwives (CPMs)** meet standards for certification by the North American Registry of Midwives. This is the only midwifery credential that requires expertise in out-of-hospital settings like home or birth center births.

- **Direct entry midwives (DM)** are educated through self-study, apprenticeship, midwifery school, or college/university-based programs that don't include nursing. Many CMs or CPMs are direct entry midwives.

- **Lay midwives** are educated through self-study and/or apprenticeships. Many are highly skilled and experienced, but they aren't certified or licensed.

Just to keep titles clear, **doulas** are present at many women's births, but they *aren't* midwives. They're experts in providing continuous support to women and families throughout labor, birth, and the postpartum period, and they can be an essential part of a woman's labor support team, but doulas aren't medically trained and aren't intended to direct medical care. See more information about doulas on pages 29–31.

Most hospital-based midwives are CNMs, and most people who use midwives deliver in hospitals. That doesn't necessarily mean that a CNM is "better" than a CM, CPM, DM, or even some lay midwives. When choosing a midwife, consider her reputation, experience, and references, just as you would with any doctor. Be particularly careful when considering lay midwives. They may be exceptionally skilled, but they haven't gone through a testing program that proves it. Anyone can say she's a midwife. If you choose a midwife with a license, you can be assured a baseline level of education. That said, I've known some lay midwives who were excellent and I've known some CNMs who were lousy. It's about the midwife more than the license.

Why choosing a midwife makes sense

The United States uses an inverted care model that's not working very well. The majority of women are perfectly healthy before, during, and after pregnancy, yet almost 92 percent see obstetricians who specialize in taking care of complex, medically risky pregnancies.[1] In other countries with far better maternal health outcomes than the United States (which ranks 60th out of 180 countries in the world), most women see midwives for prenatal care and delivery because they specialize in taking care of normal pregnancies. Studies prove this is a better model of care—midwives manage the healthy women, obstetricians take care of the sick ones. When midwives identify problems, they consult with obstetricians and, if necessary, transfer care to the higher-risk specialist.

Many women mistakenly think that a midwife may not give them the high-quality care they want. In truth, midwifery care is often more personalized, appropriate, and time-intensive and proven to reduce incidences of birth injury, trauma, and C-sections. Again, this is the model of care used in most parts of the world with the best maternal health outcomes.

Some women think that if they choose a midwife, they won't have access to pain management options like epidurals. Not true—if you deliver with a midwife in a hospital that provides standard labor and delivery care, you can absolutely get an epidural if you need or want it. The thing is, though, with midwifery care, women tend to need it less often. However, if you choose a home birth midwife or one who practices out of a freestanding birth center, an epidural is not an option.

If you have a midwife, a nurse, a partner, and a labor support team, do you need a doula?

A growing number of women are hiring doulas to assist them through labor and birth. While woman-to-woman maternity support has been around forever, doulas are relatively new. If you have a labor support partner and a nurse during labor, do you really need a doula? You might, but you want to get the right one.

There are certification and training programs available for doulas, but there aren't any regulations that govern who can and cannot say they're a doula. I've worked with some really great doulas over the years. They understand labor and birth from the physiologic and emotional angles and know how hospitals work. They're gifted at helping women get through really hard contractions and labor transitions. They understand medical language and routine procedures as well as how to help mothers work around interventions that weren't part of their birth plans. And when those plans have to change quickly, the really great doulas know how to shift gears and continue providing top-notch support. A good doula-mother relationship can be very impressive and enables many women to have the natural birth they want. Women remain more mobile, feel more supported, and use more creative coping skills to get through the toughest stretches of labor. Studies indicate that when a doula is involved in the labor process, women have fewer C-sections and report greater satisfaction with their birth experiences.[2]

I've also worked with some seriously offbeat and challenging doulas. A few have had strict personal agendas and confrontational approaches. They've started arguments with medical staff over minor issues like taking mom's blood pressure. I've known doulas who have told their clients that under no circumstances would they allow them to have an epidural or C-section. As you can imagine, this does not contribute to peace and harmony in the labor unit. I've known families who fired their doula during labor because she created too much conflict.

More often, however, doulas are kind, knowledgeable, compassionate, efficient, and supportive and a real asset to the patient and staff's overall birth experience. Some doulas also provide postpartum services for mothers and babies at home. They can help with breastfeeding and newborn care and provide other services while mom recovers from birth.

The recent increase in doula care is motivated primarily by women's desire to have more control in their own birth experiences and to avoid unnecessary interventions and C-sections. They want someone to advocate for them when their health care providers intrude on their birth plans, someone who is focused solely on their needs. I think that given the realities of labor and delivery nursing, there's definitely room on the unit for the work that doulas perform. Nurses work hard, and while one-on-one personalized patient care is their ultimate goal, they also have to do their charting, uphold hospital standards, meet other staffing needs, and adhere to a somewhat uniform care plan.

Currently in most hospitals, patients hire doulas privately, and reimbursement from insurance providers is unusual. Some hospitals are now hiring doulas on staff to provide care for select patients. Some hospitals have access to doulas who volunteer their services. Community-based doula programs often provide free or low-cost doula services for low-income women. Medicaid has begun reimbursing doulas who qualify as community health workers in Oregon, and there's hope that this may open the door for other states to be able to fairly compensate doulas.

What happens to women who can't afford a doula? They receive support from their labor nurses, their midwife or doctor, their partner, and the people they've chosen to provide labor support. For many women, that's all they need, and they report feeling well cared for.

Do you need a doula? No, you don't technically *need* one, but the right doula can be a real asset. Just make sure you check her credentials, training, and references and pick someone you feel is a good match for you and your family.

How to pick where you'll have your baby

The statistics indicate that about 99 percent of you don't really have to pick. You already know where you'll have your baby. Of all American babies, 98.6 percent are born in hospitals. That's where your doctor or midwife delivers, where your insurance covers you, and where you feel is the safest place to deliver. Plus, hospitals have the epidurals—which many women consider an absolute must. If your decision is made, feel free to skip to the next section. If you want more options or want to understand why some women make other choices, though, read on.

You have four choices when deciding where to have your baby:

1. At home
2. In a birth center located outside of and independent of a hospital
3. In a birth center located inside or adjacent to a hospital
4. At a hospital, in the labor and delivery unit

At home

The number of women making the home birth choice has been increasing since 2004. For most women who have a home birth, it is a conscious choice; they don't just deliver at home because the baby came too fast. Some choose home birth because it's affordable, or it's part of their culture, or the closest hospital is too far away. Some are afraid of hospitals, or their midwife only delivers at home. Some choose home because it offers privacy, autonomy, intimacy, and freedom, plus fewer medical interventions. Some are worried about the United States' rising C-section rate and think their best option for delivering vaginally is with a home birth.

In other parts of the world, home birth is fairly common. In the Netherlands (which has some of the best maternal health outcomes in the world), 23 percent of mothers deliver at home.[3] In developing countries, home birth is extremely common, but so are high maternal mortality rates. In India, for example, more than half of all women deliver at home, but only about half of those women have skilled birth attendants.[4] Consequently, their overall maternal mortality rate is severe: two hundred deaths per one hundred thousand live births.

That leads to the number one question most people have about home birth in the United States: "Is it safe?" That depends on the health of the mother and baby, the skill of the midwife or naturopath, access to a nearby hospital, and a good emergency backup plan. Study results vary regarding its safety, but the American Congress of Obstetricians and Gynecologists (ACOG) and the American Medical Association are against home birth. Childbirth Connection—an independent non-profit organization that provides up-to-date evidence-based pregnancy, labor, and birth information—disagrees; they say studies show *no evidence that hospital care offers clear safety benefits for low-risk childbearing families.*[5] A 2012 Cochrane Review concluded that there's no strong evidence from randomized trials to favor either planned hospital birth or planned home birth for low-risk pregnant women.[6]

Many doctors and hospital-based midwives view home birth negatively, but that may be partly because their only experience is with the women who wind up in their emergency rooms after their home births have gone terribly wrong. They don't see the majority that turn out normal, healthy, and happy. As a nurse, I understand that perspective, as well as the stress of salvaging a home birth gone awry, especially when a midwife or patient waits too long to come to the hospital for medical care. In cases (like in the Netherlands and some U.S. hospitals) where the emergency transfer from home to hospital is swift, skilled, and compassionate, however, there tends to be less trauma and better outcomes for mothers, babies, and hospital staff.

So, is home birth safe? It can be safe for low-risk, healthy women. Most women who choose home birth have a very positive experience. It's not a good choice, however, for women with medical problems or elevated risk for childbirth complications.

Side note: In the United States, you can't have a home birth *and* pain medication. It's either/or. In many parts of Europe, however, women have the option of using nitrous oxide (laughing gas) at home for safe, effective pain relief.

Birth Centers

Only 0.3 percent of American women deliver in a birth center, which the American Association of Birth Centers[7] defines as a home-like setting where care providers, usually midwives, provide family-centered care to healthy pregnant women.

There are two types of birth centers; both are considerably cheaper than standard hospital births and result in more vaginal deliveries and fewer admissions of babies to NICUs.

1. Hospital-associated birth centers are separate from a hospital's labor and delivery unit. They are usually midwife-run but obstetrician-supervised, and they cater to low-risk patients who

want low-intervention births. They offer a hybrid birth option—all the comforts of home and all the safety of the hospital, but with less intrusion, a more natural approach to birth, and a tendency to use fewer interventions. They may also offer pain management options, including IV pain medication and epidurals. They may have Jacuzzis, bathtubs, or birthing pools for water births, and birthing balls and other equipment that facilitates natural/vaginal births. Maternal and newborn health outcomes are as good as or better than those in traditional labor and delivery units, and if something goes wrong there's an obstetrician and emergency personnel available down the hall.

2. Freestanding birth centers are located outside of and independent of hospitals. They're almost always midwife-run and offer a low-invervention, vaginal "natural" birth experience. Some may offer injected or intravenous narcotic pain medication, like morphine or fentanyl, or inhaled nitrous oxide, but most do not. The safety and quality that freestanding birth centers offer is generally very good, but they vary depending on the midwife's skill, mother and baby's health, and the proximity of a hospital should things go wrong. Freestanding birth centers may be operated by certified nurse-midwives, certified midwives, and/or direct entry midwives. Check credentials and references very carefully. The advantage of using a freestanding birth center is that you'll be free from hospital-based intrusions and interventions and well supported to have a natural birth. The downside? If your birth center isn't accredited or certified and doesn't have a rock-solid emergency backup plan or your midwife isn't extremely skilled, you and your baby might not get the level of care you need, especially if things go wrong.

Are birth centers safe? According to recent studies, families who chose birth center settings in the United States experienced high-quality care with a cesarean rate (after transfer to a hospital) of approximately 6 percent. Nine out of ten mothers had vaginal births.[8] Fewer than 2 percent required an urgent transfer for either mother or newborn. The stillbirth and newborn death rates were comparable to rates seen in other low-risk populations.

Based on statistics, there's an overwhelming likelihood you will deliver in a hospital, but if you're thinking about other options, make sure you consider:

- Your health and risk level
- Your ability to tolerate pain
- Your preparation level for birth
- Your partner's feelings about where you deliver
- The qualifications of your midwife
- Proximity of your chosen place for giving birth to a hospital with a maternity unit
- Your ability to manage the details and mess of a home birth
- Certification of your birth center
- An emergency backup plan
- Access to transportation

Who's on your labor team—and how to keep your labor room drama free

We call the people who will be with you during labor "supporters" or your "labor team." "Labor coach" is old school, calling up images of a man with a whistle and stopwatch, bossing a laboring mother around. Seriously—who needs that? Women should be in charge of their own bodies during labor. They don't need to be "coached" or told what to do. They do, however, need lots of love, support, gentle reminders, back rubs, encouragement, positive affirmations, and help making decisions. Your doctor, midwife, nurses, and husband/partner are almost automatically on that team. Who else do you need to fill these roles? Probably fewer people than you think. That's why choosing your labor team carefully is really important.

Before we talk about why taking a less-is-more approach to building your labor team is smart, let me share a history lesson:

In the 1950s and '60s, the only people attending a laboring mother in the delivery room were a nurse and a midwife or doctor. Dads were relegated to the waiting room or a local bar to sit tight until the big announcement was made. Mom labored and gave birth alone (except for medical staff) with no one to support her, and dad bided his time until someone told him whether his wife and baby had survived childbirth and whether it was a boy or girl.

By the 1970s, dads were invited (or forced their way) into the delivery room, and the concept of "labor coach" was born. His job was to help mom focus, keep track of when contractions occurred (though I'd argue women didn't really need help with that), and remind her of what breathing technique to use when. His most important role was to give mom support and comfort and to be present at the moment the two of them became a family.

By the 1980s, the delivery room door had opened a little wider, and a second support person was occasionally allowed in the room. By the 1990s we had family birthing centers, and anyone mom wanted could be present. By 2000, the labor room had become crowded with friends, family, grandparents, and stepparents, and there was little room left for medical staff. Unfortunately, this was also often disruptive, embarrassing, and a bit of a zoo, as too many personalities crowded into a too-small room, sometimes trying to outdo each other in providing the best support to the laboring mother. Arguments erupted; tears flowed; yelling, screaming, and fights broke out; and in the midst of all this nonsense, a child was being born to a mother who often regretted inviting too many people to be on her labor team.

Then, one year, a horrible flu ravaged the land, and many hospitals had to shut their labor room doors to all but essential staff and one or two labor supporters, to prevent the spread of disease on the maternity ward. And peace returned to the labor room. Mothers were happier, fathers were happier, babies were healthier, and they even seemed to be born a little faster.

Where are we now? That really depends on where you're delivering, but the moral of the story is this: be very selective about who you invite on your labor team. Yours might be the perfect selection of friends and family who offer only positive vibes, loving support, and words of wisdom as your labor progresses smoothly. Or not. It could be one of those births where all hell breaks out. There could be so many people (or the wrong people) present that the intimacy of starting a family and meeting your new baby becomes diluted or disrupted. I've seen dads pushed away from mom's bed by overly eager grandparents who can't wait to get their hands on the newborn. I've seen mothers clearly humiliated when people she did not want in her room saw her naked. I've seen countless women who had no idea how to politely tell all those people to get the hell out, because all she wanted was to be alone with her partner.

So, given that it could go either way—heaven or hell in the labor room, but more likely somewhere in between—whom should you allow in?

In most families, the baby's father or your partner should have pride of place at the bedside. If he/she is ready, willing, and able to provide labor support, he/she should be the one to do that. If not, or if mom and dad want extra help, then a doula, friend, mother, sister, or other individual should be there to provide labor support.

Who else? There is no perfect number, but choose wisely, ladies— very wisely. If you let your mother in, will your husband's mother feel offended? If you let one friend in, will your other friends be pissed off? If you let in your sister who gives the perfect backrub, will your sister the chatterbox give you the silent treatment? What about dad's friends? His father? Your grandparents and stepparents? Where do you draw the line?

Ask yourself these questions:

Do you want your birth to be an intimate affair or a family matter? If you want it to be a special private moment between you and your husband or partner, don't invite anyone else. Once you crack the door to one, others will be waiting in the wings.

Do you want your birth to include significant family members? Limit your guest list to accommodate hospital rules and rules of common sense. If they're not going to be 100-percent supportive of everything you want, not willing to leave without a fuss if you ask them to, and not able to sit quietly for hours and hours; if you'd be embarrassed if they saw you naked—don't let them in.

Do you want your other children to see their sibling being born? Think this through carefully. Birth is bloody and graphic, and few children get a kick out of seeing their mothers screaming and in compromising positions. When children are well prepared, though, and mom is calm, they can handle the experience well. There's no way to know in advance how things are going to go down, so if your other children are going to be present, make sure another adult (not you or their other parent) is with them at all times, ready to whisk them out of the room if things get too intense.

If you decide to go with a larger crowd, make sure everyone knows that if at any time you want privacy or rest, there will be no questions asked and nobody gets to be huffy about it. If they can't promise they'll scoot out of the room lickety-split, fully understanding your need to change the party plans, don't invite them.

A word about fathers and partners: Obviously, mom is going to be the main focus of attention on labor/birth day, but dads and partners are also extremely vulnerable at this time. Especially if this is their first time too, they're going through a life-changing transition. They're worried about their wife or partner and their baby's health. They want to have an important role on this extremely important day. Don't invite anyone into your labor room who doesn't 100 percent get that and respect the other parent's role. And don't invite anyone who's going to try to take over this role. Nobody gets to be the other parent but that parent.

CHAPTER 3

Your Pregnant Body

Prior to becoming pregnant, you could do just about anything you wanted with your body (within reason) and could count on it to behave itself. Now that you're pregnant, that may or may not be the case anymore. Welcome to your life as a pregnant woman—aka your new normal.

What should you eat?

It was easier to be pregnant fifty years ago. There weren't any long lists of foods you couldn't eat. There wasn't any high-fructose corn syrup tripling the calorie content of common foods. There weren't as many preservatives, dyes, and chemicals in our foods. Portion sizes were considerably smaller, and having an occasional drink wasn't considered a major crime. Women ate and drank what they liked and made their own food choices. But they also lived at the mercy of their doctors, who'd unleash their wrath if the woman gained too much weight.

These days, women receive long lists of foods to avoid, foods they should eat, and vitamins they should take. In most obstetric practices, there's not a lot of focus on real nutrition education because there's usually no time to spend with patients once they've gone over the "no-no" list. That means some women don't have a clue what to eat, how much, in what combinations, and when to say when. It's no wonder, then, that record numbers of women gain way more than they should during pregnancy. Fifty, 60, even 80 pounds isn't at all unheard of, whereas back in the day, if you gained more than 25 to 30 pounds your doctor would read you the riot act. Was it patronizing? Yes! Judgmental and condescending? Definitely! But it also kept most women from gaining unhealthy amounts of weight.

When a woman starts a pregnancy at her normal weight, her body is well equipped to withstand the 30 pounds (more or less) she'll gain during a normal pregnancy. If she gains a whole lot more than that, she moves into a higher risk bracket. When a woman starts her pregnancy overweight or obese, however, her risks for high blood pressure, diabetes, and other pregnancy and birth complications go up. That doesn't mean she's definitely going to have those problems. It just means she bumps up her chances a notch or two. When she then goes on to gain way too much weight, her risks go up even further. If that woman also happens to have other health problems (called comorbidities) she dials up her risks even further.

That's the thing about food and weight gain. A certain amount of weight gain is essential for a healthy pregnancy, but too much weight gain causes big problems. It's not just about fat. It's about the integration of all your body systems with your baby's. The number on the scale is just the tip of the iceberg. There are cardiovascular and neurological implications, placental perfusion issues, musculoskeletal factors—the whole enchilada. That extra fat wraps around your vital organs, travels through your blood vessels, and is stored in seriously unhealthy places. One reason obese women have more C-sections than normal-weight women is that they have fat stored around the muscles and tissues around their vagina—a fat blockade that babies can't always get past. Unfortunately, too many women learn about this too late in the game.

OK, now that I've been scary, let's talk specifics. You'll be given a list of foods to avoid eating during pregnancy because they're associated with increased risks for complications for some women. Following is what the Department of Health and Human Services, Office of Food Safety says that pregnant women should avoid, why, and what to do.

DON'T EAT THESE FOODS	WHY	WHAT TO DO
Soft CHEESES made from unpasteurized milk, including Brie, feta, Camembert, Roquefort, *queso blanco*, and *queso fresco*	May contain *E. coli* or *Listeria*.	Eat hard cheeses, such as cheddar or Swiss. Or check the label and make sure that the cheese is made from pasteurized milk.
Raw COOKIE DOUGH or CAKE BATTER	May contain *Salmonella*.	Bake the cookies and cake. Don't lick the spoon.
Certain kinds of FISH, such as shark, swordfish, king mackerel, and tilefish (golden or white snapper)	Contains high levels of mercury.	Eat up to 12 ounces a week of fish and shellfish that are lower in mercury, such as shrimp, salmon, pollock, and catfish. Limit consumption of albacore tuna to 6 ounces per week.
Raw or undercooked FISH (sushi)	May contain parasites or bacteria.	Cook fish to 145°F.
Unpasteurized JUICE or cider (including fresh squeezed)	May contain *E. coli*.	Drink pasteurized juice. Bring unpasteurized juice or cider to a rolling boil and boil for at least 1 minute before drinking.
Unpasteurized MILK	May contain bacteria such as *Campylobacter*, *E. coli*, *Listeria*, or *Salmonella*.	Drink pasteurized milk.
SALADS made in a store, such as ham salad, chicken salad, and seafood salad.	May contain *Listeria*.	Make salads at home, following the food safety basics: clean, separate, cook, and chill.
Raw SHELLFISH, such as oysters and clams	May contain *Vibrio* bacteria.	Cook shellfish to 145°F.
Raw or undercooked SPROUTS, such as alfalfa, clover, mung bean, and radish	May contain *E. coli* or *Salmonella*.	Cook sprouts thoroughly.

continued

DON'T EAT THESE FOODS	WHY	WHAT TO DO
Hot dogs, luncheon meats, cold cuts, fermented or dry sausage, and other deli-style meat and poultry	May contain *Listeria*.	Even if the label says that the meat is pre-cooked, reheat these meats to steaming hot or 165°F before eating.
Eggs and pasteurized egg products	Undercooked eggs may contain *Salmonella*.	Cook eggs until yolks are firm. Cook casseroles and other dishes containing eggs or egg products to 160°F.
Eggnog	Homemade eggnog may contain uncooked eggs, which may contain *Salmonella*.	Make eggnog with a pasteurized egg product or buy pasteurized eggnog. When you make eggnog or other egg-fortified beverages, cook to 160°F.
Fish	May contain parasites or bacteria.	Cook fish to 145°F.
Homemade ice cream	Homemade ice cream may contain uncooked eggs, which may contain *Salmonella*.	Make ice cream with a pasteurized egg product safer by adding the eggs to the amount of liquid called for in the recipe, then heating the mixture thoroughly.
Meat: Beef, veal, lamb, and pork (including ground meat)	Undercooked meat may contain *E. coli*.	Cook beef, veal, and lamb steaks and roasts to 145°F. Cook pork to 160°F. Cook all ground meats to 160°F.
Meat spread or pâté	Unpasteurized refrigerated pâtés or meat spreads may contain *Listeria*.	Eat canned versions, which are safe.
Poultry and stuffing (including ground poultry)	Undercooked meat may contain bacteria such as *Campylobacter* or *Salmonella*.	Cook poultry to 165°F. If the poultry is stuffed, cook the stuffing to 165°F. Better yet, cook the stuffing separately.
Smoked seafood	Refrigerated versions are not safe, unless they have been cooked to 165°F.	Eat canned versions, which are safe, or cook to 165°F.

Will these foods definitely cause you to have complications? Probably not in most cases. But because we have scientific data demonstrating that these foods increase risks for complications in *some* mothers, you're going to feel like crap if you indulge and "something happens."

I ate lots of Brie and fish with all of my pregnancies (back in the day when we were only advised to avoid coffee and alcohol), and so did generations of women before me. I didn't know they were a problem, but if I had, I probably would have abstained. I was practically perfect about adhering to the dietary advice of the times with my first pregnancy, but coffee crept into my second one, and I was a regular consumer in pregnancies three and four. I made my own peace with it, and as those babies turned out just fine, I figured a cup of joe after a long sleepless night was OK.

I'm not a fan of food hysteria and across-the-board mandates that say because a few women might be affected by these foods, all women should avoid them. The problem is, we can't always know who is going to develop problems and who isn't, so we make recommendations for everyone. I can say this: if you are one of the few who should absolutely not have eaten that sliced ham, you're going to feel a whole lot of guilt and regret, and that feels worse than almost anything.

Now, let's create a better list of all the things you *can* eat:

- Feel free to have unlimited amounts of fresh veggies and, as long as you're not diabetic, plenty of fruit.

- Make sure you eat enough lean protein from a variety of sources like chicken, turkey, beef, pork, tofu, beans, eggs, nuts, and, yes, some fish.

- Try to have some protein with every snack and meal. That keeps you from getting hungry too often and keeps your blood sugar balanced.

- Go for whole grains like brown rice, whole wheat, oats, barley, quinoa, and others. Choose whole grains over refined and processed ones every chance you get. Whole grains have more nutrients, are digested more slowly, and will keep you full longer.

- Drink water (not soda) and, if you can digest it, milk. If you can't drink milk, get your calcium from fortified orange juice and calcium-rich foods like tofu, leafy greens, and fortified grains. If all else fails, take calcium supplements to keep your bones and your baby's strong.

- Eat healthy fats such as olive oil, many vegetable oils, avocados, nuts, and nut butters. Other fats will occur naturally in certain foods like meats and dairy products. Aim for the lean stuff and avoid fried foods, but don't go fat-free. Your body and your baby's need fats for many metabolic and developmental reasons. Just choose them wisely.

OK, that's the basis of your healthy pregnancy diet. How *much* do you need to eat? Not much more than you ate prepregnancy. It only takes about 500 extra calories per day to support a pregnancy. That's an orange, an egg, and a glass of milk. It's a turkey sandwich with not much mayo. It's a medium-sized broccoli, chicken, and rice bowl. It's two Snickers bars or one milkshake. It's one fried cherry hand pie.

Does that mean you can't ever enjoy a donut or a late-night Häagen Dazs bar? No, it does not. You're entitled to an indulgence every now and then. You're pregnant, and it's silly to think you're going to have the willpower of a runway model all the time. But don't make it a daily habit to chow down on fried chicken and waffles, and don't start thinking you're eating for two. Yes, technically you are; that doesn't mean you get to eat double the calories.

What about coffee and alcohol? We don't really know what levels of either are safe for pregnant women. Women who drink alcohol heavily during pregnancy dramatically increase the risk of their child's being born with fetal alcohol syndrome, which affects the child physically and mentally for life. It's total bad news and not something any mother should ever do to her child.

That said, I know my mom knocked back a martini or two once in a while during her pregnancies, and my siblings and I are all bright enough. I know that women in other countries are sometimes encouraged to have a little wine to relax or help digestion, so why in the United States do we tell pregnant women to abstain 100 percent?

Because we don't know how much booze is safe for any particular woman. We don't know which woman will report having had only one beer when in fact she's an alcoholic who can't stop at one. Health care professionals don't want to give a woman permission to use her own judgment and then get sued when she delivers a damaged baby.

Same with coffee. We don't *think* babies will suffer complications if mom drinks a cup or two. But if she's a caffeine junkie who guzzles espresso shots all day, frankly, we don't know exactly how that will affect her baby. And we don't want to be the one standing in court saying, "I told her a cup was OK."

This is where we need a heavy dose of common sense. If you're really going to commit to doing the absolute best thing for your baby, don't eat junk food or any of the other processed "food-like substances" with the endless ingredient lists your grandmother wouldn't recognize. Don't drink alcohol and coffee. Don't touch any nonorganic food, and don't drink anything other than crystal spring water as pure as virgins in May . . . But if that seems over the top to you, then use your own judgment and do the best you can. The research is out there. The do-not-eat lists are well known. Make your own decisions about what you put into your body, knowing full well what history has shown us, what science has taught us, what medicine will tell us, and what your baby needs.

How to deal with feeling like crap

The first trimester of pregnancy is rarely much of a party. Sure, you may be happy as hell to be pregnant. You might be excited, relieved, delighted, and astounded. But if you're like 50 to 90 percent of newly pregnant women, you also feel like crap. You're sleepy, exhausted, queasy, and weepy. You're so tired you can barely make it home from work without taking a quick nap in a parking lot. You're hungry, but you can't eat. You can smell the contents of someone's lunch box across the street and the contents of your laundry basket from two blocks away.

Why do so many women feel lousy during the first few months of pregnancy? Because the pregnant body is undergoing a complete overhaul that's ruled by unfamiliar hormones. Pregnant women go through a lot during the process of creating a new human being. I firmly believe the reason most of us feel so nauseated is because we're growing somebody else's brain in our bellies. This is not easy. This is incredibly complicated and demanding work. It's also incredibly cool and magical but at least for the first few months, this work makes many women feel gross, at least until most of the early cell division is out of the way. Once they've adjusted to their new hormones and gotten past the first 12 to 16 weeks, most women get a reprieve and feel pretty good for a few months. About 15 to 20 percent of women continue to feel queasy through their entire pregnancy and that totally sucks. The majority of women, however, think that the second trimester and most of the third feels A-OK.

Now, for those of you still in that first trimester, let's figure out how to get through the day.

Before you go to bed at night, make sure you have a package of crackers at your bedside along with a glass of water.

First thing in the morning, before you even get up to pee, munch on a couple of crackers, sip just enough water to swallow them, and then wait a few minutes before you do anything else. This gives your stomach a chance to wake up without revolting.

Throughout the day, munch on bland foods (or anything that sounds good to you) frequently. Try your best to eat before hunger strikes. Pack snacks in your purse so you don't ever have to wait for something to eat.

Don't worry about eating a balanced diet during the early yucky weeks. Eat whatever you can stomach. In a perfect world, that would be organic and plant- and lean protein–based foods, but the first trimester is not a perfect world. In fact, plants and protein are often the foods that gross out pregnant women the most. That makes sense from an evolutionary standpoint. Back before women had long lists of foods to avoid, nausea and food aversion potentially prevented pregnant women from eating poisonous plants and potentially tainted meats. It was a protective mechanism that probably kept developing fetuses alive. Even though most of us live where safe food sources are abundant, our bodies haven't gotten the memo, and they're still protecting us from eating hemlock and rotten eggs. If all you can eat is white toast, well then, eat white toast. Just go with it.

Many women find they can tolerate these foods during early pregnancy:

- Miso soup
- Chicken broth
- Mashed or baked potatoes
- Ginger tea
- Lemonade
- Cereal
- Crackers
- White rice
- White or wheat bread
- Raw fruits and veggies
- Sour foods and citrus fruits
- Yogurt and ice cream

You'll want to totally avoid anything that is:

- Greasy, smelly, gassy, spicy, or slimy
- Loaded with sugar, chemicals, and artificial ingredients
- Proven to make you gag on sight
- On the official "don't eat during pregnancy" list (even if that's all you want to eat)

Every now and then, when you're not feeling too sick, try eating something you enjoyed before you started feeling sick all the time— not chips or a box of donuts, but something that's actually good for you and your baby, like broccoli or chicken and rice or tabbouleh. Little by little, you'll feel like eating again, and when you do, make it healthy.

Now, how about that fatigue? You know the cure—sleep. Don't beat yourself up about not having the energy you used to have. Don't tell yourself you have to stay awake, have to keep going, have to push on. Instead, take a nap. Lie down. Put your feet up. Feel like going to bed before sunset? Go for it. Your body is busy doing the most important work it has ever done. Our bodies heal and grow and do the huge job of getting a baby ready for the world during sleep and rest. Just honor the cues your body sends you.

How can you get the rest you need while still working or taking care of your other children or going to school? That depends on how supportive your boss, coworkers, family, friends, and teachers are. Ask for support. If your other kids are too little to cut you any slack or if resting at work isn't going to happen, then give your day job (or kids) all you've got. When you get home from work (or your partner gets home and you can hand off childcare duties), forget about cooking dinner; order takeout (or make it a cereal supper). Don't even think about vacuuming your bedroom or attacking the clutter or doing anything else. Just rest. Go to bed early. Conserve your energy for the obligations and responsibilities you can't get out of, and leave everything else off your to-do list. First on that list is being pregnant. Second, taking care of your kids and job. Third—don't bother; you're going to be too tired to do anything else for a couple of months.

Once you've figured out a few things you can eat without hurling, and you've come to terms with just how much rest and sleep you actually need, then add one more thing to your "how not to feel like crap" regimen—exercise. It's essential for helping your body create the healthy blood vessels and nerve synapses you need to grow a great placenta and have a healthy pregnancy. It's even more important in the early months than ever. Frankly, I think this is a design flaw in Mother Nature's pregnancy plan, because most women just want to tuck in under a down comforter and wake up sometime around week 16. I want you to do what you can, however, to get some exercise every day. Take a walk, go for a swim, or hit the elliptical trainer for half an hour (or even ten minutes!). After that, go tuck in under that comforter with your crackers and ginger ale. Believe me, most of you will feel pretty good, pretty soon.

What if you're in that 15 to 20 percent who don't feel better after the first few months? Check in with your health care provider regularly and make sure you don't have any underlying health issues going on. If you can't keep any food down, you may need medical attention and maybe even a prescription. Hyperemesis gravidarum is a serious complication of pregnancy that causes severe nausea and vomiting. It can lead to dehydration, miscarriage, and cardiac complications. Some women have it so bad they have to be hospitalized for IV hydration, antinausea and vomiting medication, and even tube feeding to get nutrition into their body while bypassing the stomach.

Here's the bottom line for the first trimester when you feel like crap: It's normal. Take care of yourself. Take it easy. Eat what doesn't make you barf, and keep your eyes on the prize—the second trimester, when almost every woman feels pretty darn good.

What about sex?

For most women, sex during pregnancy is a great big "Yes, please!" It's safe, it's fun, and all that extra blood flow to the lady bits and pieces makes them more sensitive and raring to go than ever. That is, unless all those extra hormones, weight gain, and fatigue make you feel gross and unattractive, or you're in the small subset of women who would be happy to partake in a romp but have been told by their health care providers to abstain.

Let's tackle the "yes, please" crowd first: Once the green fog of morning sickness subsides, many women report that sex during pregnancy is some of the best sex of their life. They credit super-sensitive skin, a new level of intimacy with their partner, and a new appreciation for their body. Plus, there's no worry about trying to get pregnant or trying not to get pregnant, which means sex can be all about fun and not about function. As long as you don't have any health problems that make sex risky (we'll cover those later; see page 51), there's no reason why you can't have as much sex as you want for as long as you want. You may reach a point during the last few weeks when sex is awkward due to your big belly, but if you're still in the mood, be creative. Go for it as long as you want to, and stop when you're not into it anymore.

I often get asked if baby can tell you're having sex. Frankly, no one has ever gotten a straight answer on that from an actual baby, but we suspect they're entirely unaware of it. Remember, even if the cervix gets bumped during sex, the baby is well protected, floating in fluid and nowhere near the playing field. Even if your partner is being extremely, umm, "enthusiastic," the odds of your baby being aware are very slim.

I also get asked why your uterus or abdomen gets tight and hard during sex, especially during and after orgasm. It's because your uterus is contracting mildly in response to sex. This isn't the kind of contraction that causes cervical dilation, though. You wish, right? If that were the case, nobody would mind going through labor.

Can sex make labor start? Well, maybe, if labor was already imminent and all it needed to get started was a nudge. Hormones in semen called prostaglandins can help the cervix soften and become ready for labor. It's not as effective as a big old dose of Pitocin, though it's a heck of a lot more fun, at least for the guy.

Can sex start preterm labor? For a very small percentage of women whose cervix is unable to remain closed, sex could start preterm labor. That's not likely to happen unless the cervix and uterus were just looking for an excuse to get things started. As a good safety rule, if you have nonpainful contractions after sex, drink some water and rest a while. They'll probably go away. If they continue or they're painful, give your health care provider a call. Don't be shy. Tell him or her you had sex. Believe me, they won't be shocked. They get this call all the time, and it's no big deal.

How about those women for whom having sex sounds about as appealing as licking the bottom of a pond? That's normal, too. Some women want nothing to do with sex during pregnancy and want to keep their body to themselves. They're tired, nauseous, achy, uncomfortable, heavy, bloated, irritable, and constipated—and frankly, none of those adjectives are synonymous with hot sex. If this sounds like you, don't push it. If you're not into it, you're not into it, and there's nothing wrong with you. Tell your partner to be patient and you'll find your way back to sexy-time eventually.

One woman wrote and said as soon as she became pregnant she couldn't stand the smell of her husband. It wasn't a hygiene issue or something he was eating. She just hated his smell, and she didn't want to have sex with him. Another woman told me her boobs were so sore she didn't want her boyfriend to hug her, much less fondle her. One woman told me she felt sorry for her husband, who wasn't used to going without, so she tried having sex, but the jostling made her so nauseated, she barfed. After that, he was happy to wait a few months until she felt better. Don't worry if sex isn't your thing for a while. You've got a lot going on, and that's completely normal.

How about women on the "no sex" list? Certain complications make sex potentially dangerous for some pregnant women. These include:

- Placenta previa (the placenta is covering the cervical opening)
- Abnormal vaginal or uterine bleeding
- Active herpes lesions
- Sexually transmitted infections (STIs)
- Ruptured amniotic membranes
- Cervical incompetence
- A history of premature labor
- A prematurely dilated cervix
- An undiagnosed abnormal discharge

For some of these women, "no sex" means nothing goes in the vagina, but it's still safe to engage in other sexual activities, including masturbation and oral sex. For others, no sex means nothing, nada, zilch, fugettaboudit. Nothing vaginal, nothing anal, nothing oral—no sex. They can take care of their partner's needs, but sexual stimulation and orgasm could cause enough uterine/cervical irritation and contractions to cause trouble.

How will you know if you're on the "no sex" list? Your doctor or midwife should tell you explicitly, but she may also use vague terms like "pelvic rest" or "abstinence." If you're not entirely clear what that means for you, don't be shy: speak up and ask.

How many women are on that list? Not many. The exact number is unclear, but it's a small one. For most of you, feel free to go for it— or not.

What if your partner is worried about hurting you during sex? Have him or her read this section and if that's not enough to put his or her mind at ease, have a frank discussion about what feels good, what feels like "too much," and reassure your partner that you'll let him or her know if anything hurts. If they're still too concerned and want to abstain while you're pregnant, that's their prerogative. Respect his or her right to say "not now."

Just how tough is your baby? Dealing with fears about exposure to drugs, alcohol, cigarettes, and other toxins

Pregnant women aren't super keen on talking about the recreational drugs they take, the alcohol they drink, and the cigarettes they smoke during their pregnancies. There's lots of guilt and judgment associated with all that. They're more OK with talking about exposure to chemical fumes and environmental toxins. Regardless of how they're exposed, most mothers who either knowingly or unknowingly dose their babies with something potentially damaging feel frightened. They all wonder the same thing: Is their baby going to be messed up?

There's no way to answer that question with complete assurance. Few babies are conceived, carried, or raised in perfect environments, and most turn out just fine. Most mothers don't knowingly drink, smoke, or do drugs during pregnancy, but some do. In fact, prior to the 1960s (when word first got out that fetal exposure to alcohol and tobacco was bad), many mothers who smoked and drank kept it up throughout their pregnancies, and their babies were usually fine. It's only been in the last fifty-some years that we've focused on reducing exposure. Pregnant women today not only have to avoid obvious toxins, but they're also given a long list of potentially dangerous foods and substances to avoid. Women are worried about nail salons and hair dye, blue cheese and lunch meat, pollution, a sip of champagne, and fumes emitting from cheap furniture. They're scared about black mold, paint fumes, lead chips, electromagnetic fields, and so many unknown and potentially dangerous components in our environments, it's a wonder any pregnant woman ever gets any rest! But most babies are born healthy, normal, and ready to take on the world. Most. A few, admittedly, are born with serious problems. But because there's virtually no way to eliminate *all* exposure, my recommendation is that you avoid what you can and try not to worry too much.

Babies are very resilient and very fragile. They're protected from a lot and absolutely vulnerable. What one baby can tolerate, another cannot. I've seen babies born addicted to heroin or prescription painkillers who've gone through withdrawal like total badasses. Sure, they had symptoms, nasty ones, but they recovered. I've also seen babies born addicted to cigarettes who suffered severely when their nicotine supply was cut off. I've seen babies born to mothers who drank a glass of wine daily throughout pregnancy who turned out just fine, and babies born to mothers who drank the whole bottle daily who will be impacted for life. Babies of mothers who smoke pot turn out very differently from babies born to mothers who smoke methamphetamines. It all depends on the toxin, the extent and duration of exposure, and what stage of pregnancy it occurs in. A toxin that's tolerable to one baby may be completely destructive to another. I think every baby deserves the best possible chance in life, which means developing with the least amount of toxic exposure.

What about exposure to chemical fumes or other environmental toxins—for instance, chemicals in the workplace, pollutants, or cleaning solutions? Most babies turn out just fine. We don't know, however, precisely what causes some babies to develop learning, behavioral, or social disorders, and there's growing concern that some may be related to toxic exposures. We're living—and growing our babies—in a world that's chemically loaded and technologically altered, and we're seeing more children diagnosed with ADD, ADHD, ASD, and a host of other disorders. We don't know why some children become autistic, violent, depressed, or dysfunctional. Could it be the chemicals and drugs?

We honestly don't know because we can't directly study the effects of chemicals, drugs, and toxins on pregnant women and babies. It's dangerous, illegal, unethical, and simply not done.

What do you do if you've exposed your embryo or your fetus to something bad? Stop the exposure! If it's drugs—quit taking them. Cigarettes? Quit smoking them. Booze? Put down the bottle. Chemicals in your house? Go outside, ventilate the place, and stay somewhere else until the air has cleared. Is your workplace toxic? Ask for a cleaner workspace. Believe me, nobody thinks any of this is simple, but it has to be done. The sooner you stop the exposure, the sooner your baby can recover.

Should you tell your doctor/midwife about your exposure? In a perfect world, the answer would always be "yes!" If exposure is related to a legal substance, then by all means, tell your doctor or midwife so he or she can help you and your baby.

What if we're talking about drug or alcohol exposure? Talking to your health care provider about substance abuse during pregnancy can create some particularly tricky situations. Many docs and midwives do drug tests as a routine part of prenatal care, so your drug use may not actually be a huge surprise. But here's the tricky part. While a good health care provider can be an excellent resource for substance abuse recovery services, some providers are bound by law to take action or file a report with Child Protective Services (CPS) when they know their pregnant patient is drinking or using drugs. Others use more discretion and may direct their patient to resources without blowing a whistle.

When a woman is open and honest about needing help, she should be treated with compassion and support. But a woman who admits to substance abuse during pregnancy is often treated to stern judgment. Her admission can place her in legal hot water if she lives in a state with punitive drug and/or reproductive health laws. In some states, women have had their newborns removed from their custody for as little as testing positive for marijuana. Other states are more lenient even with heavier drugs, especially for women who are actively pursuing sobriety and getting help.

The legal implications of asking for health care assistance with addiction should be at the bottom of a pregnant woman's list of worries; the health and well-being of her baby should be at the top. But addiction takes that list and tears it up. It's too complicated a problem to be viewed as black or white, good or bad. It's addiction. There's nothing simple about it. If you can't stop using without formal support and a rehab program, the best thing you can do is to ask your doctor for help, regardless of the legal implications. Your health and your baby's development are the most important things. Do what you have to do to eliminate the toxins that may damage your baby's health, even if that means opening yourself up to judgment.

Just how tough are babies? Pretty tough. So are most mamas. But some babies aren't tough at all, and some mamas need more help than others. In a perfect world, any type of exposure would be dealt with compassionately and a mother's fears would be relieved. If only we lived in a perfect world.

Common medical bumps in the road

Spotting, discharge, miscarriage, and ectopic pregnancy

Among the topics I get the most emails about are early pregnancy spotting and weird discharge. Is that because most women have these conditions? No, but it's common enough, usually normal, a bit disconcerting, and sometimes downright frightening.

If you're in your first trimester and notice a bit of spotting (pink, brown, or red bleeding, but not enough to soak a pad) or reddish-brown discharge, your first reaction is likely to be fear. That makes total sense: before you became pregnant, any sign of blood meant you were having your period—that is, not pregnant. However, even if you have a little spotting while pregnant, the odds are in your favor that you're still pregnant and your pregnancy is still normal. Spotting during early pregnancy does not necessarily indicate a miscarriage.

As noted earlier, between 20 and 30 percent[2] of women have some spotting during early pregnancy, but only about half of those "spotters" miscarry. The other half are experiencing either cervical irritation, implantation bleeding, or hormonal changes, or they're eliminating old blood from the cervix.

Cervical irritation is caused by increased blood flow directed to the uterus that allows it to nourish and grow a baby. The cervix is loaded with tiny blood vessels that are filled with that extra blood. They can break easily and release a little blood—say, if they're bumped during sex, if there's an infection brewing, or often for no good reason anyone can determine.

If spotting happens right after sex, that's probably what caused it. The cervix got nudged and bumped, and that was all it took to leak a little blood. It's most likely coming only from the cervix, not from the uterus, and in most cases it's not an indication that you have to avoid sex. But because any kind of spotting is likely to freak you out, you may feel more secure if you limit the bumping and nudging for a while and engage in alternative activities.

If spotting is associated with itching, burning, a gunky-funky discharge, or vaginal/labial pain, let your health care provider know. Those are all signs of a vaginal infection, which calls for a trip to your doctor or midwife's office and a prescription. Since you're pregnant, don't try and self-diagnose or treat this with an over-the-counter medication until you've chatted with your health care provider.

Implantation bleeding can happen between the fourth and sixth weeks of pregnancy. The fertilized egg has finished traveling through the fallopian tube, found its way to the uterus, and burrowed into the uterine lining. (From there you'll grow a placenta, an umbilical cord, an amniotic sac, and a 7- to 8-pound baby.) Sometimes implantation causes a bit of spotting.

If your cervix is simply reacting to the roller coaster of hormones rocketing through your bloodstream, there's nothing you need to do about it. You'll adjust sooner or later. It doesn't indicate anything's wrong. It's just your body's way of figuring out what it's doing.

Very often, there's no telling what causes spotting. It generally goes away on its own and never points to any problem that's brewing. Wear a pad so you can keep track of how much bleeding you're having, and give your doctor or midwife a call to let her know about it. She may want to see you in the office, take a peek with the ultrasound, or draw blood to determine how high your pregnancy hormone (human chorionic gonadotropin, or hCG) levels are, but she may also tell you to hang out and see what happens. That's because chances are good nothing's wrong that requires medical attention, but also because, if you are having a miscarriage, there's not much she can do in the very early weeks to stop it. Again, about 15 to 20 percent of all pregnancies end in miscarriage, most before the woman even realizes she's pregnant. The other 80 to 85 percent don't. A trip to the midwife or doctor won't change those statistics, but it may provide you with reassurance that you're doing just fine.

Here's the most impractical advice I'm going to give you in this book: Try not to worry too much about spotting (yeah, right). The odds are in your favor.

Spotting that turns to bleeding or comes with pain is entirely different. It still may be nothing to worry about, but you may be experiencing a miscarriage or an ectopic pregnancy.

Miscarriages occur for lots of reasons, but they usually boil down to one of three things. One, something was wrong with the embryo or fetus and nature decided to halt production. Two, something is off-kilter with your hormones and they weren't able to maintain the pregnancy. Three, something's wrong with your cervix and it's not able to retain the pregnancy.

If you have one miscarriage, you and your doctor will most likely chalk it up to the first reason—a faulty embryo or fetus. If you have more than one miscarriage, it's time to investigate other causes.

Miscarriages are confirmed by the amount of bleeding that occurs, by ultrasound, and/or by blood tests that indicate the hCG levels are declining. Most miscarriages resolve themselves through bleeding and cramping that expels the embryo and what's called the "products of conception." Sometimes, however, women need either medicinal help (a prescription) or a medical procedure called a D&C (dilation and curettage). Since your provider has already been alerted that you're bleeding, he or she will evaluate how you're doing and make that decision with you. If you're seeing a midwife and you need a D&C, you'll probably be referred to an obstetrician to do the procedure.

If your bleeding is caused by an ectopic pregnancy, you will probably experience big-time cramping and maybe one-sided abdominal pain. An ectopic pregnancy happens when the fertilized egg gets stuck or tries to implant in the fallopian tube instead of the uterus. The tube isn't flexible enough to accommodate a growing embryo. Pain happens as the tube stretches, and if the developing embryo remains stuck, it will eventually rupture. This is painful, dangerous, and potentially life-threatening; it requires medical care. That's why a phone call to your provider is important whenever you see blood during pregnancy.

Ectopic pregnancies are diagnosed by ultrasound, and the sad news is that an ectopic pregnancy isn't going to make it. An embryo can't survive in the fallopian tube, and the only way to prevent a ruptured tube and potentially great harm to the mother is to terminate the pregnancy. This can be done either with a prescription that halts cell division and creates a miscarriage or with surgery. We don't always know what causes an ectopic to occur, but we do know that it sometimes happens when the tube is scarred from previous infections. Will it happen again? That depends on a lot of factors, like the condition of that tube after an ectopic pregnancy and the condition of the other tube. Though the chance of having another ectopic is higher, most women never experience a second one, and more than 50 percent of women go on to have a healthy pregnancy. It's a tragedy when it does occur, but it's not something you're likely to repeat.

Bacterial vaginosis

Bacterial vaginosis is another topic that's at the top of my email list. That's because women often find out they have it only when they're pregnant or having trouble getting pregnant. They've heard it can increase miscarriage, and they're pretty freaked about it.

Bacterial vaginosis[3] (BV) is caused by an overabundance of normal vaginal bacteria. The vagina is home to lots of bacterial colonies that are healthy when they live in harmony with each other. Under normal conditions, they keep each other in check and everybody gets along just fine. If something occurs, however, that knocks them out of balance, like the introduction of foreign bacteria via sex or the disruption of one colony due to antibiotics, or for some unknown reason, then other bacterial colonies reproduce like crazy. Then the cervix and vagina may become irritated or develop a funky, stinky discharge. Just as often, though, women have no clue there's trouble brewing down below until they find out they have BV during pregnancy or when they have a Pap smear or vaginal culture during a well-woman exam.

Usually, BV goes away by itself without treatment. The body's immune system figures out what's going on and mounts a peacekeeping mission to regain bacterial harmony. If the immune system is out of whack, however, because of health issues like an autoimmune disorder, an unhealthy lifestyle, smoking, an imbalance in vaginal pH, or some other situation (sometimes including pregnancy), the woman's ability to heal herself may be compromised. If BV really gets out of control, it can travel up the vagina through the cervix and into the uterus, which can inhibit fertility or compromise an otherwise healthy pregnancy. This doesn't happen very often; most of the time, when BV is diagnosed, antibiotics are prescribed to kill the overdominant bacterium.

Is BV a sexually transmitted disease? Not technically, but sex can be a contributing factor. Women who have multiple sex partners tend to develop BV more than others; women are also more susceptible to BV when they are pregnant, even if they are monogamous.

I regularly get emails from women who say they have taken antibiotics (sometimes more than one course) and still have BV. I recommend they look closely at their diet, stress level, and lifestyle to determine what else they could do to support their immune system. Our body is designed to heal itself; when it's unable to do that, it's often because we're sabotaging our own healing process. Take probiotics. Clean up your diet. Ditch the smokes (that's a must when you're pregnant, anyway). Dial down the stress. Examine your life and lifestyle and find ways to fine-tune your self-healing mechanisms. Oh, and talk to your doctor or midwife to find out if they have any suggestions about how to create bacterial harmony in your most intimate body part.

Prenatal Tests

Testing, testing, one, two, three . . . For millions of healthy mothers around the world, prenatal testing for maternal and fetal health problems is unheard of, uncommon, or unavailable. For American women, it's routine, seemingly endless, and often the focal point of prenatal care. Let's find out what's essential and what's optional for women to have the healthiest pregnancies

What are all those prenatal tests for, and do you really have to have them?

Prenatal care for *healthy* women includes an endless list of lab, ultrasound, and monitoring tests—blood tests, urine tests, screening tests, diagnostic tests, genetic tests, fetal monitoring tests, cervical tests—and that's just for women with normal pregnancies. Women with health complications have an even longer list. What are all those tests for, and do you really need all of them? Do they all contribute to maternal/fetal health, or are some done for medical-legal defense purposes? What happens if you opt out of all or some? Are there negative consequences to any of these tests?

Most women never ask these questions. They go to their prenatal appointments and take the lab slips and test orders their doctor hands them without ever asking what they're for. They stick out their arm (or expose their belly) and try not to wince when the needle goes in. Or they lie on an exam table, pull up their shirt (or take off their pants), and watch in wonder as an ultrasound reveals the mysterious little one growing inside. Then, at their next appointment (or, over the phone), their doctor or midwife tells them if any of the tests were abnormal or if they need further discussion.

Because the doctor or midwife orders the tests and receives the results, it never occurs to many women to take ownership of the process. They figure their health care information will be given to them on a need-to-know basis, and they'll just follow orders. This is a big mistake.

The prenatal tests that *are* important for every pregnant woman are those that can indicate or rule out significant conditions that may directly affect her or her baby's health. But not all prenatal tests are required or even necessary. In fact, some are completely optional. Some are done just to cover all the bases; some are done to protect the doctor or midwife. Some routine tests may even unnecessarily alter the course of a pregnancy. So instead of ordering everything on the menu, many women would be wiser and better served by ordering à la carte.

Prenatal testing breaks down into three categories: routine, screening, and diagnostic.

Routine tests

Routine tests are done on most pregnant women because abnormalities detected through testing can significantly impact both the mother's and the baby's health. Plus, most of the conditions tested for have treatment options that are usually (though not always) effective.

Which *routine* tests are important for most pregnant woman?

- A complete blood count (CBC) to test for anemia

- Blood typing (including Rh screen) to find out if your blood is type A, AB, B, or O (super important in case you hemorrhage and need a transfusion) and whether you're Rh+ or Rh– (super important to prevent Rh incompatibility, which can cause dangerous complications for your baby and future pregnancies)

- Rubella screen for immunity to rubella (aka German measles; if you contract it while pregnant, depending on the trimester, there is a risk of miscarriage or stillbirth, and a range of severe health problems for babies who survive)

- Hepatitis panel for hepatitis A, B, or C (a virus that causes inflammation of the liver and can be transferred to baby during birth)
- Pap smear to test for cervical cancer and human papillomavirus (HPV)
- Syphilis test (for a sexually transmitted disease that can damage babies)
- HIV test for the virus that causes AIDS (if you're HIV positive, receiving treatment during pregnancy can prevent mother-to-child transmission in 99 percent of cases)
- Cystic fibrosis screen, to determine if you are a carrier (an optional genetic test that's best done prepregnancy)
- Glucose tolerance test to screen for gestational diabetes, which can cause abnormal weight gain and other complications for mothers and babies and glucose imbalance for newborns
- Urine analysis and culture, plus frequent urine dips to rule out infection, diabetes, and preeclampsia
- Group B strep test for bacteria that can transfer to babies in the birth canal and cause respiratory infections in babies; mothers who test positive receive antibiotics during labor

Ultrasounds are routinely performed to determine fetal age, size, and well-being, but they aren't absolutely necessary for every woman. Some women get one, some have several, and although they're generally considered safe (ultrasound waves don't seem to cause fetal harm when used for short periods of time by professionals), they sometimes deliver results that may unnecessarily alter the course of the pregnancy. We'll talk more about this later in the chapter.

Screening tests

Screening exams look at several different factors before determining results. For example, genetic screening evaluates results from a blood test and the patient's age and ethnicity and estimates the chances for having an abnormality. These tests do not diagnose a problem; they only signal whether further diagnostic testing should be done.

Screening exams that are offered to all pregnant women include:

- Pap smears, to check for the presence of abnormal cervical cells that might indicate cervical cancer

- Urine dip tests to check for abnormal glucose (sugar) levels that may indicate diabetes

- Urine dip tests to check for increased protein that may indicate preeclampsia

- Blood tests during the first trimester and second trimester, for genetic screening (quad screen is a blood test/ultrasound combo) to determine a baby's chances of having genetic anomalies

Diagnostic tests

Diagnostic tests go further than screening tests. They look at patients with increased odds for having a problem and determine what that problem is. For example, if a pap smear (screening exam) finds abnormal cervical cells, then a biopsy (diagnostic exam) will determine what kind of cells they are and whether the woman has cancer. If a urine dip indicates increased glucose, diagnostic tests will find out if she has diabetes. Similarly, if a genetic screening test indicates higher than average odds for having a baby with a problem, then a diagnostic test like chorionic villus sampling or amniocentesis will usually determine for sure if an abnormality is present and what that abnormality is.

Diagnostic tests include:

- Chorionic villus sampling, done between 10 and 13 weeks of pregnancy. It involves removing a small amount of the chorionic villi (wispy placental projections) from the placenta and sending it out for genetic testing. The procedure is done by either inserting a needle through the abdomen (guided by ultrasound) or passing a small tube through the vagina and cervix.

- Amniocentesis is done between 15 and 20 weeks of pregnancy. It involves inserting a needle (guided by ultrasound) through the abdomen and into the amniotic sac. Fluid from the sac, which contains fetal cells, proteins, and fetal urine, is removed through the needle and sent to a lab for genetic testing.

We're going to cover screening and diagnostic genetic testing in more detail later in this chapter. But no matter which test is ordered, no matter how routine, every patient should understand what she is being tested for, why a test is needed, how results could affect her health, and what happens next. Some of you may be thinking, "I don't want to bother my doctor with too many pesky questions. I don't want her to think I don't trust her." Here's what I say: Health care providers don't know what you need to know unless you ask them. They don't own your health; you do. They're not in charge of your health; you are. They work for you. You hire them and pay them for information. It's your body, your baby, your health, and your health care. *Ask the questions.*

What about ultrasounds?

Here in the United States, ultrasounds are considered a routine part of prenatal care. They're so common that even women who don't technically *need* an ultrasound for medical reasons expect to have one so they can get a glimpse of their baby before he or she is born. Ultrasounds are useful for screening out abnormalities, locating the placenta, determining how many babies are in the uterus, guiding medical procedures (like amniocentesis and chorionic villus sampling), identifying fetal age and size (more or less), and determining the baby's gender. They're also lots of fun and provide photos that are cute as heck, but they're not mandatory for all mothers in order to ensure a healthy pregnancy. Millions of women around the world have healthy babies without ever having an ultrasound.

Are there any reasons why you *shouldn't* have an ultrasound? Yes. Ultrasounds are generally safe and usually accurate, but they're not exact. In fact, in some circumstances, they can give faulty information, with serious consequences.

For example, in the case of a woman who doesn't know the date of her last menstrual period and therefore doesn't have a precise due date, a first trimester ultrasound can do a fairly good job of determining fetal age and a target date for delivery. It's not as accurate for that purpose in the second or third trimesters, though; in fact, it can be off by a couple of weeks. This presents problems when a doctor/midwife uses an inaccurate due date determined by a late ultrasound to schedule an induction. If the woman isn't actually due (because her ultrasound was inaccurate for dates—very common), her induced labor may not progress properly. That puts her at greater risk for having a C-section and a preterm baby.

Sometimes an ultrasound is the perfect tool for detecting problems before they become a crisis. During the last weeks of Angela's pregnancy, her belly stopped getting bigger and her baby became less active. Her midwife consulted with an obstetrician, who ordered electronic fetal heart monitoring and an ultrasound procedure called a biophysical profile, which measures baby's heart rate, muscle tone, movement, breathing, and the amount of amniotic fluid surrounding the baby. Angela's tests indicated her baby was stable, and another checkup was scheduled in a few days. When that ultrasound indicated the baby was less active and her amniotic fluid levels were greatly diminished, Angela was admitted to the hospital for further monitoring. Her midwife and doctor agreed that an induction of labor was probably a good idea, and when the baby was born (vaginally), they were relieved they'd made that decision. A knot in the umbilical cord had reduced blood flow between the placenta and Angela's baby. That hadn't been visible on the ultrasound, but the test did provide valuable information that led to Angela's admission to the hospital and early delivery of a healthy baby.

But ultrasounds also may contain a small potential for risk. Ultrasounds are sound waves, a form of energy that transmits directly into your baby's delicate and developing tissues. Although they've been used for decades, and they're considered overwhelmingly safe when performed by professional technicians for the shortest time possible, there are some concerns about the heat that ultrasounds generate. No large-scale studies have determined a direct connection, but some experts are concerned that the heat caused by excessively prolonged or repeated ultrasounds could be connected to increased rates of autism. Studies[1] conducted on mice have indicated significant changes in fetal neurons after prolonged ultrasound exposure. Ultrasound concerns date as far back as 1982, when the World Health Organization reported, in its summary "Effects of Ultrasound on Biological Systems,"[2] "animal studies suggest that neurological, behavioral, developmental, immunological, haematological changes and reduced fetal weight can result from exposure to ultrasound." I think the important thing to focus on here is that ultrasounds are safe when they are not excessively prolonged or repeated. When performed by professional technicians, ultrasounds are rarely prolonged or repeated too often.

I don't think there's any reason to freak out about one or two medically necessary ultrasounds. They're not likely to cause any problems. I wouldn't however, choose an ultrasound just for fun. Use some common sense: get one if you need one, but don't opt for extras, and don't be concerned that you're missing out on excellent prenatal care if your health and pregnancy are so normal that your doctor or midwife says you don't need one at all.

The pros and cons of genetic testing

It used to be that only women at high risk for having a baby with a genetic anomaly were offered genetic testing. Women who had a previous baby with a birth defect or multiple miscarriages, mothers over thirty-five, and women or their partners who were known to carry chromosomes for genetically acquired disease were encouraged to do these tests. If a problem was diagnosed, they'd have the option to continue or terminate their pregnancy. As gene testing has become more sensitive and sophisticated, it's become available at earlier stages of pregnancy and in some cases can be done less invasively. Now all women, not just the high-risk ones, are offered genetic screening tests.

Very early during prenatal care you'll be presented with genetic testing options. If you're not paying attention, you may not realize you're having a genetic screening test done, especially if it's lumped in with other tests being ordered. If your health care provider is doing his job, however, he'll break the tests down so you can be an active participant in the decision of whether or not to do genetic testing. If your provider doesn't spell things out in a way you completely understand, then ask, ask, ask.

Many parents opt out of genetic screening. They may be concerned about the minor risks involved. Some don't want to know if their baby will be born with genetic or health problems and are fine with accepting the baby with whatever issues he or she may have. That's the way it was for all parents prior to the 1930s. It's the way it still is for most parents in the world who have limited access to health care.

In the previous section, I explained the difference between screening and diagnostic tests. The American Congress of Obstetricians and Gynecologists (ACOG)[3] explains it like this:

Screening tests are performed during pregnancy to assess the risk that a baby has certain birth defects, including Down syndrome, trisomy 13, trisomy 18, and neural tube defects. The following screening tests may be offered:

- **Maternal serum screening**—measures the level of three or four substances in the mother's blood. It's performed during the second trimester to assess whether the baby is at increased risk of Down syndrome, trisomy 18, abdominal wall defect, and neural tube defects.

- **First trimester screening**—combines the results of a special ultrasound test called nuchal translucency screening and blood (serum) tests (PAPP-A and hCG) to assess whether the baby is at increased risk of Down syndrome, trisomy 21, trisomy 18, and other chromosomal disorders.

The information received from screening tests is usually reassuring, and mothers go on with their pregnancy feeling good that their baby is healthy or normal. If screening exams indicate increased odds for problems, though—for example, a genetic abnormality like Down syndrome or spina bifida—then the parents have to decide whether or not to do further tests. As mentioned already, a screening exam doesn't indicate for sure that a baby has one of these problems, just whether the baby has a greater than normal chance of having the problem.

Once parents hear their test results, they have to decide how comfortable they are with the information they've received. If the odds are higher than normal, they have to decide on next steps. At this stage, many parents decide they'll accept the odds and won't do anything further. They just want a baby, any baby, even a baby who may or may not have problems. Many parents, however, need to know for certain whether their baby has a problem. They'll need diagnostic tests, which will either reassure them that their baby is fine or confirm that their baby is not fine.

If it's determined their baby has a serious problem, parents have to make a really hard decision—to continue the pregnancy knowing their baby will be born with a health problem or to terminate the pregnancy. This is one of the most difficult choices that any parent can face.

As of this writing, doctors can screen for around two thousand specific genetic problems. How often are these tests right? Though the tests keep getting more sophisticated and accurate, they catch only about 80 to 95 percent of abnormalities (depending on the test), with a 4- to 6-percent false positive rate. That means they won't catch 5 to 20 percent of genetic problems, and sometimes they'll indicate problems where there really aren't any.

There are no right or wrong answers when it comes to genetic testing. Ask the questions and talk about what test results would mean to you and your family. Then make an informed decision and be prepared to deal with the results. The only wrong answer comes from not asking the questions.

Nonstress tests, biophysical profiles, and other late-pregnancy tests

If you're having a moderate-risk to high-risk pregnancy, you may be wondering if the testing will ever end. Most women won't need anything other than the routine stuff that happens at every prenatal appointment, but some will need a more thorough look-see. They may need additional ultrasounds, kick counts, fetal heart monitoring, contraction monitoring, and even an amniocentesis. These tests should be done only on an as-needed basis and are certainly not necessary for every mother. If your doctor recommends one, you know what to do: ask questions. Find out why it's recommended and how it will change your pregnancy or care. If all is well and you and your baby aren't having any complications, you really don't need the extra scrutiny, which sometimes results in unnecessary interventions—opt out. If there are solid medical reasons why you and your baby need extra attention—go for it. Here's what you can expect:

- **Contraction and fetal heart monitoring**—This is a noninvasive (meaning nothing goes into the body) test to watch for contractions and see how the baby's heart reacts. This might be ordered if you're having regular contractions before 37 weeks, if your baby isn't moving normally, if there are health concerns regarding your baby, or if you're close to your due date and your doctor/midwife wants to know if you're in labor. It requires two elastic straps and two external monitoring devices—one to detect contractions and one to record baby's heartbeat. These monitors, which look like round discs (about the size of the top on a take-out coffee cup), are held on your belly by the soft straps. They're attached to cables that connect to a computerized monitoring device. The information detected is printed on a paper monitoring strip and displayed on the computer screen. A nurse and your provider read the strip by looking for specific patterns, which helps them evaluate whether or not you're in labor and how your baby is faring. The amount of time you're monitored may be as short as 20 minutes or could be longer, depending on how long it takes before your provider is reassured that all is well or decides other interventions need to take place.

- **Nonstress test**—Very similar to contraction and fetal heart monitoring, this noninvasive test is done during some pregnancies that are past 28 weeks gestation. Nonstress means that it does nothing to cause stress (aka contractions) to the baby. Nonstress tests are done to evaluate how baby is doing under normal conditions and how its heart reacts to its own movements. This may be done if mom is past her due date or isn't feeling the baby move as much as usual, if there are concerns about how the placenta is functioning, or if mom has any other medical conditions that could affect baby's well-being, like diabetes or hypertension. It generally takes about 20 to 30 minutes to place the monitors and record enough fetal activity to establish that all is well. The nurse and provider are looking for specific heartbeat patterns that generally indicate baby's heart and brain and the placenta are A-OK. They want to see the heart rate vary from beat to beat and increase in response to movement. If baby is sleeping during monitoring, though, there may not be enough activity to produce the specific patterns that indicate well-being. In that case, the nurse might give you a glass of juice or water to stimulate baby to wake up, or she might place a buzzer that makes an annoying noise against your belly. That usually wakes baby up.

- **Contraction stress test**—This uses the same monitoring techniques as the nonstress test, but with "stress" (aka contractions) added. If a patient having a high-risk pregnancy is close to her due date and the doctor wants to be certain the placenta can deliver adequate oxygen to the baby during contractions, that's when a contraction stress test might be done. Mom will be monitored and an IV will be started. She'll receive Pitocin through that IV to generate contractions; then she and baby will be monitored to determine whether or not baby tolerates contractions well. The nurse and provider will be looking for specific heart rate patterns that generally indicate fetal well-being. They'll also look for the absence of heart rate slowing (called decelerations) after contractions. If they don't see any decelerations and they do see a normal amount of accelerations (baby's heart speeding up), it is considered a negative test and all is presumed to be well. This test may be done as part of an induction or to make certain that mom and baby are both OK to continue with a pregnancy. It's kind of old-school and not performed as commonly as it used to be (primarily because other tests, like a biophysical profile, provide adequate information in a less cumbersome and invasive way).

- **Biophysical profile**—This test is a two-part combo, one part fetal heart monitoring and one part ultrasound. Your provider may order it if she can't get enough information from a nonstress test, if a nonstress test isn't reassuring, or if she's worried about specific issues going on with your baby. She'll do a basic nonstress test and then follow it up with an ultrasound that looks for these five things in your baby:

  1. Heart rate
  2. Breathing movements (baby practices breathing in the uterus)
  3. Body movement
  4. Muscle tone
  5. Amount of amniotic fluid

Each of these is evaluated on a 2-point system. A final score of 8–10 is considered reassuring. A 6 is equivocal, which means they can't tell if baby is OK or not. A score of 4 or less means more testing needs to be done and/or the baby needs to come out.

- **Amniocentesis**—Earlier in pregnancy amniocentesis is done for genetic testing purposes. Late in pregnancy, it's done to determine fetal lung maturity. If there are indications that a baby should be delivered early but there's concern that a baby might not be mature enough to breathe on her own or could develop respiratory distress syndrome after birth, then a provider might do an amniocentesis.[5] He'll measure the surface-active properties of surfactant phospholipids secreted by the fetal lungs into the amniotic fluid. The test involves the same procedure as earlier in the pregnancy (a needle is inserted through the abdomen and into the uterus and amniotic sac and fluid is withdrawn), but this test takes only a few hours to return results. Amniocentesis is sometimes done in combination with two injections (24 hours apart) of steroids to mom to stimulate fetal lung maturation. If your doctor is recommending a late-pregnancy amniocentesis, than you almost certainly have medical concerns that warrant it. I wouldn't opt out of having this procedure—unless your doctor can't give you any good reason for doing it, and this is rare. If you don't understand fully why an amniocentesis is ordered, then keep asking questions until you're comfortable with the answers.

- **Kick count**—If a baby isn't moving as often as usual or if mom can't tell if baby is moving, a kick count provides a simple way to either provide reassurance or let mom and her provider know she needs more evaluation. Mom can do this test on her own at home whenever she wants or as often as her provider recommends. All she needs to do is have a snack or a glass of juice, lie down on her side, and start counting. The goal is to record 10 kicks, rolls, movements, bumps, or nudges within two hours. If she feels all 10 in 5 minutes, all is well. As soon as she feels 10, the test is done. If she doesn't feel 10 within two hours (or less), she should contact her physician, who will probably advise her to go to the hospital for a nonstress test.

Most of the time these tests come back with reassuring results. Sometimes they simply lead to more testing. Occasionally, however, they send a signal that baby needs to be delivered. That's what these tests are for—to determine which babies need help and which are just fine.

Prenatal Education
and Birth Plans

The more you know about pregnancy, labor, and birth, the better prepared you'll be to deal with them, whether your experience is straightforward and wrinkle-free, or way more challenging than anticipated. A comprehensive parental education also makes it easier to construct a realistic, totally usable birth plan. As I mentioned in the introduction, information really is the key to everything.

Getting a prenatal education—before and beyond what the hospital teaches

Prior to the 1950s (and still today in many parts of the world), the only education a woman received about her impending labor and birth was what her mother, sisters, doctor, midwife, or friends told her. Most women simply did what came naturally without having the benefit of a specialized curriculum. There weren't any six-week sessions of evening lessons or weekend intensives. There weren't dozens of books, magazines, and websites devoted to all things childbirth related. For most women, childbirth education consisted of watching your siblings being born or the cow deliver her calf.

When formal childbirth education programs began, they were considered as essential as prenatal care, but they were also focused primarily on having a natural, family-centered birth. They were the answer to the overly medicalized, isolated birth experiences common in hospitals prior to the 1970s natural childbirth movement. For decades thereafter, women took classes with their labor coaches to learn how to relax, breathe, change positions, and do all they could to facilitate a birth sans medication and surgery. These classes and the natural childbirth movement were damn successful, too. From the early 1970s through the 1980s, women and their partners gained a measure of control over their births. Many of the unpleasant and potentially humiliating and even dangerous practices of shaving, enemas, and episiotomies were greatly reduced. Women were no longer knocked out, strapped down, and delivered by forceps with their husbands off in the waiting room (or a bar). We gained a lot of traction in those years, as doctors and hospitals acquiesced to what women wanted.

The American birth culture has changed a lot since then, and women today have different issues to deal with. Having a baby nowadays is loaded with medical-legal standards, technology, interventions, tests, monitoring, anesthesia, decisions, plans, goals, and a bevy of birthing philosophies. That's why women need a good prenatal education—to learn how to navigate the medical system and negotiate for the birth they want and the one that's safest for them. When women don't have a clue how the birth industry operates (pun intended), they end up with more interventions than they need or are safe. Thus we have the highest C-section and NICU admission rates in history.

When women get prenatal education, most take classes recommended by their health care providers and delivering hospitals. They may do courses online or start classes during their second or third trimester to learn the ropes of a standard hospital birth. They'll learn basic birth anatomy and physiology and about coping with contractions, medical procedures, pain management, and medications. They may learn a few tips in case they want to go natural, but with fewer than 40 percent of women having their babies without an epidural, there's no longer such a big emphasis on natural childbirth. They'll learn what an epidural is and get a tour of the birthing rooms and nursery, and they will be encouraged to write up their birth plan. What they won't get is a comprehensive education about all the birthing options available. They won't be schooled on how to have a safe home birth or the value of using a birth center. They probably won't learn about the wide variety of natural pain management techniques that range from Lamaze to Leboyer to HypnoBirthing to Birthing from Within to Orgasmic Birth to . . . (yeah, Orgasmic Birth—that's a thing).

If, like most U.S. women, you're planning on having an epidural, why do you need to know about all those other options for labor and delivery management? A good prenatal education is important for every parent, not just the ones aiming for natural childbirth, because having a baby is loaded with complications brought on by the overmedicalization of what should be (for most women) a fairly straightforward and normal body function. Even if you want an epidural and aren't planning on doing anything on the natural childbirth list, you need to know what's normal, what's not, how to cope with the unexpected, and what to do about the pain if the anesthetist is busy (yes, this happens).

Getting a good prenatal education doesn't mean you have to choose between having an all-natural birth and having an all-medical birth. It means you go into labor with your eyes open, fully aware of how things work. It means you've explored your options and are equipped to make your own health care decisions. It means you have the information you need to have the birth you want, whether that includes an epidural or a birth tub, oxytocin, or nitrous oxide.

So how do you get a well-rounded prenatal education? Sign up for the class recommended by your health care provider, but be aware that different providers and practices have different focuses. Midwife-centered practices tend to offer a more comprehensive education program that covers birth as a normal physiologic process. Obstetrician-centered practices tend to funnel patients into the hospital's curriculum, which, as already mentioned, may focus on medications, hospital procedures, and anesthesia options. After you take those classes, check out books from your library that cover other options. I really like HypnoBirthing (a method pioneered by Marie F. Mongan, with practitioners and courses for expectant mothers) because I think they offer the most usable information on how to accomplish a low-intervention birth. I also think Lamaze has a lot to offer. They've evolved from the early days of strict breathing patterns. I like some of what the Bradley and Grantly Dick-Read methods have to offer, though I think they're a bit strict and tend to characterize hospital staff as the enemy (which they're absolutely not).

Learn everything you can and create your own childbirth education program. Somewhere along the way, you'll realize what you want your birth to be like. You'll bond with certain tips and discard others. You'll figure out what works for you and what goes out the window. You'll gather enough information to make well-informed choices during your birth experience. Remember, you're in charge of your health care, and your physician is your partner, not your boss. The more you know, the better equipped you'll be to be a good partner in your own birth.

How to determine whether you want your birth to be all natural, all medical, or something in between

Some women are 100-percent sure they want an all-natural birth. No medications, no epidurals, minimal time in bed, maximum time on their feet, in a tub and using a birthing ball, and absolutely no C-section. Other women know for sure they want all the bells and whistles the hospital has to offer. If they could get an epidural during their last week of pregnancy, they'd be all for it. If they end up with a C-section, no problem. They want the full-meal, medical deal. Most women fall somewhere in between, though some never give it any thought. Their plan is to do whatever their doctor or midwife says and to follow orders.

If you aren't already leaning strongly toward either a natural or a medicalized birth plan, here's how to determine what you want. Give yourself a comprehensive prenatal education, as described in the preceding section. Take into consideration your health history, medical conditions, your partner's preferences, your providers' recommendations, and your options for where to give birth. Then go with your gut and remain flexible.

You probably already know if you have a high pain tolerance and a high level of trust in your own body's ability to function normally.

Those are going to be huge factors in how you approach your birth. I know a few women who are scared to death to approach labor without medical experts at their bedside. I also know women who are terrified that if they deliver in a hospital all the staff will be out to get them. Most of the women I know, however, aren't that nervous, and they're fine with a middle ground approach.

Going into labor set on a rigid all-natural, or an all-medical, or a following-orders birth plan isn't such a great idea, because labor and childbirth rarely go exactly as planned. Every birth is a previously untested navigation between one mother's body and one baby's body, and babies never consult birth plans. Instead, I recommend women approach labor as naturally as possible and then adapt as needed. That's why it's important to learn what's involved in births that veer away from your preferred birth plan.

Even if you want an epidural, you should learn how to relax and breathe into contractions, get into positions that facilitate labor, and participate in decisions made about your birth experience. In many hospitals, you can't get an epidural until you're about 4 centimeters dilated, and you might have to wait until an anesthetist is available. That could mean hours of contractions you'll need to cope with. Even if you're planning an all-natural birth, you need to know about other pain management options available at your birth facility in case you change your mind mid-labor. Believe me, that happens a lot.

I think the best birth style and plan is this: Aim for a natural birth with the least amount of medical intervention whenever possible. Be flexible. Trust your body and your health care providers and go with the flow. If everything goes as planned, excellent; but if plans have to change, so be it.

How your pregnancy determines your birth plan

As your due date approaches and you're preparing and planning for the birth of your dreams, it helps to think back over your pregnancy. If you've had a high-intervention, heavy-duty medically oriented pregnancy, it may not be realistic to think that you'll give up all the medical stuff on the day you go into labor so you can have an all-natural birth. On the other hand, if you've had a perfectly normal pregnancy without a lot of fuss and bother, it's probably realistic to plan on a low-tech, low-intervention birth. Likewise, if you've been happy to follow along with everything your provider has recommended throughout your prenatal care, chances are you'll be happy with her recommendations for labor and birth, too. As goes your pregnancy, so goes your birth—to an extent.

Let's say your birth plan includes delivering at home with a midwife and a doula. If you're healthy and in a low-risk pregnancy category, and you have a rock-solid emergency backup plan, chances are everything will go as planned. Add on a getting-to-know-you meet-and-greet with your midwife's backup OB and a tour of the local hospital, and you're all set.

Let's say your birth plan includes an unmedicated vaginal birth at the hospital. If you've established prenatal care with a health care provider who has a good reputation for supporting natural births, plus you're healthy and educated about natural pain management techniques, chances are good you'll achieve your dream birth. But what if your provider isn't all that supportive? What if you've gained a ton of weight and your blood pressure is too high? What if you haven't studied so much as a whiff of deep breathing and relaxation techniques? What if your pregnancy has been one crisis after another? Then I'd say, don't get too bonded with your natural birth plan. Your pregnancy doesn't bode well for that kind of birth. I'm not saying it's impossible. I'm just saying your pregnancy hasn't led you down that path so far.

What if you want a low-intervention birth, but you have a few medical conditions that required a lot of testing and extra health care? What if you've been worried all nine months about something dangerous happening to you or your baby? What if you can't go a week without calling your provider about one worry or another? There's nothing wrong with any of those things, but you should realize that a stressful, test-heavy, high-intervention pregnancy may well be followed by a similar labor and birth.

I know a woman who is a self-described hypochondriac. If she hears about someone with a weird disease, she's convinced she has it, too. When she got pregnant, she was certain she'd be among the one in a bajillion women whose baby had a third hand. She opted for every test in the book and couldn't fully relax even when she was told her baby was perfectly normal. When she felt a little queasy and heard about hyperemesis gravidarum, she was sure that's what she had (she didn't). When she got a mild headache, she was convinced it was preeclampsia (it wasn't). She was ready to sign on the dotted line for every potential complication. She knew she was being a little nutty, but she couldn't help it. Being sick was her thing.

The crazy part was that despite all the unnecessary medical tests and false alarms she had during her pregnancy, she seriously thought that she'd be able to have a completely natural labor. But the minute labor started, she was sure the cord was wrapped around the baby's neck or his heart would stop beating. She didn't dare hang out at home during early labor; she insisted on being admitted to the maternity department when she was only 1 centimeter dilated. She never felt secure enough to let go of the fetal monitor, walk the halls, take a bath, or try other techniques that facilitate a normal birth. It shouldn't come as a surprise that when her baby's heart rate dipped a wee bit (and then quickly returned to normal), she freaked out and insisted on an emergency C-section. Her doctor didn't think she really needed one, but this patient couldn't relax and let things happen naturally. Sure enough, before long, she was in the operating room having surgery. When it was over, she was disappointed she hadn't had her natural birth, though she was the only one who had ever thought that was a possibility.

If you want a low-intervention birth, your best bet is to aim for a low-intervention pregnancy. If you don't need tests and treatments, opt out. If you need extra medical attention, by all means get it, but then recognize that you may need extra medical attention during labor, too. Again, that doesn't mean a low-intervention birth isn't possible. It just means you're already under the microscope. Prepare for the birth you want, stay flexible, and go with the flow.

Birth plans: pros, cons, reality checks

Here's what I love about birth plans: their intent. I love that parents carefully consider their options and create a plan. I love how birth plans provide evidence that a couple has thought through what they want their birth to be like. They demonstrate to medical staff that this mother and her partner have educated themselves, have some preferences, and are good communicators. Birth plans signal to health care providers that these parents want things *their* way, not just the routine way. A plan makes everyone involved in a birth pay attention a little more closely and go about things a little more deliberately.

Here's what I hate about birth plans: how some couples think of them as contracts rather than goals or wish lists. Because it's unreasonable for couples to mandate what will and won't happen "no matter what." I hate when a birth plan shows that a mother and her partner are rigid, unwilling to consider anything that might not be reflected in their birth plan, and that they're approaching their birth ready to fight. Birth plans can make parents come to their births with fear and hostility.

I've seen all kinds of birth plans, from the funny to the hostile, and the birth plans I like best are the ones that fall somewhere in between. A good birth plan includes a mother's preferences for pain management, the type of birth she prefers, the interventions she hopes to have or avoid, what she likes and dislikes, and any specific issues she'd like us to know about. It should also include which procedures she'd like done or not done to her baby, whether or not she wants to breastfeed, and any cultural, spiritual, or religious practices that are important for us to know about and respect. If there are siblings, we love it when a birth plan mentions how the parents would like us to introduce them to the baby or incorporate them into the birth experience. A good plan sets the intention and tone for the birth they hope to have, but doesn't set it in stone. Instead, a good plan is open and flexible, much like mothers have to be when they give birth.

Birth plans that demand certain conditions be met and specific interventions be avoided, or present a list of dos and don'ts that must be adhered to, are unrealistic and hard to achieve. Here are some examples:

Under no circumstances will an IV be inserted in mother or baby at any time.

Really? There are no circumstances when an IV would be OK? What if mom is bleeding to death and needs emergency surgery? What if baby contracts an infection and needs antibiotics? When you put it that way, most mothers would say, "OK, fine. Under those circumstances, an IV would be OK."

Believe me, we get it that many mothers don't want routine IVs during labor. In most cases, we're fine with that, but we need at least a little wiggle room. When a birth plan instead says, "We'd prefer not to have an IV inserted during labor or in our baby after birth unless there's a strong clinical reason," that's a lot easier to accommodate and shows that parents get it. Sometimes emergencies happen and you need an IV.

No epidural or pain medication is to be offered or administered under any circumstances.

Really? Not even if mom is begging us to give her some relief? Not even if she's used up all her breathing, relaxation, and natural coping techniques and she still has hours and hours of labor ahead of her? Not even if she desperately needs a C-section? Not even if she's screaming at us to "give me the f***ing epidural NOW!"

Most first-time mothers have no idea what they're really going to be dealing with during labor. They write their birth plan with a good idea that labor is going to hurt. What they don't really get is that for most mothers, it's incredibly intense, it's the worst pain they'll ever experience, it goes on for hours, and it can become unbearable if labor doesn't move quickly.

It's not that hospital staff doesn't support natural birth or believe women when they say they want to have a natural birth. We do. We see it happen every day, and we love it. Many mothers, especially first-timers, come to labor with every intention of going without pain medication or an epidural and then change their minds when the rubber meets the road. They hadn't figured on labor being that painful. And because a dose of drugs in the IV is readily available—and if that's not enough, an epidural is generally just a phone call away—many mothers who come in with all-natural plans end up having epidural births. These mothers are not wimps. It's just that they need another option for coping with the pain, and here in the United States we don't have many options. It's kind of all or nothing. They're offered IV narcotics or epidurals or nothing at all. That's about it. In other countries—like the United Kingdom, Australia, most of Europe, and many other parts of the world—women can opt for nitrous oxide (laughing gas), which provides a safe middle ground between natural birth and epidurals. Nitrous oxide takes the edge off the pain well enough that a much lower percentage of women who use it opt for an epidural. With nitrous oxide, they just don't need it. (See more on page 135.)

Most hospitals in the United States don't have birthing tubs available either. If every woman had the option to soak in a nice hot bath during labor and use some laughing gas if she needed it, our epidural rate would drop like a stone.

When you're writing up your birth plan, stay open and flexible. Tell your hospital staff what you're hoping for and ask for their support in achieving your goals. Then go into labor with the best of intentions and lots of preparation, but don't kick yourself if you switch gears. The interventions offered at the hospital are tools that are available if you need them. Don't rule any of them out, because labor is hard work and you might just need a few tools to get the job done.

How to Deal with Late Pregnancy Curve Balls

This won't happen to all of you or even to most of you. But for those of you who reach the last few weeks and find your doctor/midwife talking about an issue that seems like a total game changer, this is for you.

You can see your birth plans going up in smoke, and you're rattled. What are you supposed to do now? That depends on what the curve ball is, but whenever something comes flying at me from out of the blue, I either duck and cover, bat it to the outfield, or wait for the next pitch. Unless you're having a really big emergency, a curve ball doesn't have to be a game changer. It may, however, require a few new strategies, a negotiator, or some new teammates. Let's break down a few common curve ball scenarios.

Your doctor says your baby is too big and wants to schedule an induction or a C-section—what now?

This happens so often it makes me want to scream. It's more common in doctors' than midwives' offices, because midwives tend to be less intervention oriented. They trust the normal physiologic processes of birth. They do fewer inductions, and they don't do C-sections at all. If a patient needs a C-section, midwives transfer care to an obstetrician.

Here's how this curve ball often gets pitched: A woman is a few days or weeks shy of her due date. Her doctor measures her belly and says, "This baby's getting too big. I don't think we'd better let you go much longer, or it's going to be too big to fit through your pelvis. Let's get you on the schedule for an induction." Maybe the doctor orders an ultrasound to estimate fetal size and weight (which can be off by a couple of pounds, give or take); maybe he doesn't. By suggesting the baby is too big, he plants a seed of doubt in the mother's mind. Some doctors forgo the induction suggestion altogether and tell mom there's no way she'll be able to push out a baby this size, so she needs a C-section. Now mom thinks she needs surgery before she's even given her body a chance to do what it's designed to do.

Estimated fetal size is rarely a good reason to do an induction or C-section, especially when a baby's not due yet. Even the American Congress of Obstetricians and Gynecologists agrees on this. Mothers of all sizes have been delivering small, medium, and large babies vaginally without being induced for thousands of years. There's no reason why this generation of mothers are incapable of delivering their babies. Yes, some mothers with gestational diabetes do grow very big babies, but most mothers don't have that condition, and even those who do deserve the benefit of the doubt that they're capable of having a vaginal birth. They need support, confidence, and encouragement, not seeds of doubt, early inductions, and/or surgery.

When mothers are supported to go into labor naturally, they're far more ready, willing, and able to deliver whatever size baby is inside. When labor is induced, however, before a mother's body is ready to give birth, she often fails to dilate, her labor doesn't progress, and far too often she winds up in surgery for a C-section. I can't tell you how many inductions and C-sections for "too big" babies end up delivering perfectly normal-size babies.

If your doctor tells you she wants to induce or do a C-section because she thinks the baby is too big, tell her you don't want either. You'd rather wait for labor and see what happens. If after going through labor it turns out she's right and you need a C-section, well then, so be it. Most of the time, though, spontaneous labor that's allowed to progress normally results in a normal vaginal birth. Don't let that seed of doubt grow. In most cases, our bodies know what to do to get our babies out.

Your ultrasound shows you have too much/ too little amniotic fluid—what now?

Too much amniotic fluid is called polyhydramnios. Too little is called oligohydramnios. They're very different conditions, so we'll break them down separately.

Polyhydramnios (too much fluid) happens in only about 1 percent of pregnancies. For most mothers diagnosed with this condition, it resolves itself and doesn't cause problems. For some, however, polyhydramnios is associated with serious complications. The March of Dimes says these include premature birth, premature rupture of membranes, placental abruption, stillbirth, postpartum hemorrhage, and malposition of the baby.[1] About half the time, nobody knows what causes it. In the other half, it can be attributed to birth defects that affect a baby's ability to swallow (which helps regulate amniotic fluid levels), maternal diabetes, Rh incompatibility, twin-to-twin transfusion in identical twins, problems with the baby's heart rate, or an infection in the baby.

When a doctor suspects polyhydramnios, she'll order an ultrasound to measure the volume of amniotic fluid in the uterus. If it's only mildly elevated, she'll probably take a wait-and-see approach and schedule another ultrasound in a week. If there's a lot, she might order a more detailed ultrasound or other tests to look for causes. If she can fix the problem, through medication or diabetes management, then she'll continue monitoring to make sure baby remains well. Or she might order an induction of labor to get the baby out before bigger problems develop.

It's important to remember that this condition is pretty rare; it often resolves on its own without treatment and doesn't cause fetal complications in most cases. Sometimes, however, it's serious. This is something you need to determine with your doctor. Ask lots of questions, and make sure you fully understand your individual circumstances and risk factors. If you need an induction, so be it. That's what they're for—to get at-risk babies out of at-risk mothers before something really dangerous occurs.

Oligohydramnios means there's too little amniotic fluid in the uterus. It happens in around 4 percent of pregnancies. If it happens during the first six months of pregnancy it can indicate bigger problems than if it happens in the last three months. About 12 percent of women who go two weeks past their due date will develop oligohydramnios.

Your doctor/midwife might suspect oligohydramnios (which is confirmed by ultrasound) if you're not gaining weight, or your baby isn't growing properly, or you're leaking fluid. If "oligo" happens early in your pregnancy, your doctor might want to check for fetal birth defects of the kidneys or bladder, maternal diabetes, or high blood pressure. It can also be caused by maternal dehydration and by certain medications that regulate the amount of fluid in mom's blood vessels. Oligo that occurs early in pregnancy is associated with miscarriage, premature birth, and stillbirth.

Oligo occurs naturally once your water has broken and, assuming that happens before or during labor and near your due date, it's no big deal. If it occurs late in pregnancy but your membranes are intact, the biggest complication is that there might not be enough fluid to keep the umbilical cord floating freely. Without fluid to act as a cushion, the cord can get pinched or compressed, which restricts blood flow, nutrition, and oxygen from mother to baby.

Sometimes, all that's needed to fix the problem is to regulate mom's medications, have her drink more fluid, recommend she rest a bit more, and/or schedule follow-up ultrasounds and wait and see. If the fluid level remains low or is getting worse, and/or if the baby is showing signs that she's being negatively impacted, an induction might be a good idea. Again, that's what inductions are for—to get babies out before they get into trouble.

If oligohydramnios occurs during labor and fetal heart monitoring indicates that the cord is being affected (which shows up as a fetal heartbeat that's either too slow or too fast), that can sometimes be fixed with an amnioinfusion. A tube is threaded through the cervix and into the uterus. An IV saline solution is infused through the tube to add fluid back into the uterus to protect and cushion the cord.

If your doctor says you have oligohydramnios, make sure it's diagnosed through ultrasound. Ask questions. Find out if a wait-and-see approach is a good idea or if your baby is developing problems. Then go with what feels safest to you. If you need to deliver before you go into spontaneous labor, so be it.

You've tested positive for group beta strep—what now?

Group beta strep (also called group B strep, beta strep, or GBS) is a naturally occurring bacterium that lives in the vagina, rectum, nose, throat, and other mucous membranes. It's no big deal for the 25 percent of mothers who carry these bacteria in the vagina as part of their normal bacterial flora. It's potentially a huge deal, however, for babies who get infected with GBS at birth, because it can cause sepsis, meningitis, and respiratory infections. Early onset infections in newborns usually occur during the first week after birth. Late onset infections can occur up to three months after birth.

Since GBS does not make most women sick, they don't know whether or not they're carrying it and could potentially transfer it to their vulnerable newborn. That's why all women receiving traditional prenatal care are screened for GBS at 35 to 37 weeks gestation. If they test positive, they'll need to receive IV antibiotics during labor to prevent transmitting the bacteria to their baby at birth. It's important for women to know that this is *not* a crisis, sickness, emergency, or game changer. Except for the fact that they have to get an IV during labor (and most women who deliver in hospitals have one anyway) and receive antibiotics approximately every four hours, it's kind of no big deal. It doesn't change a woman's ability to have a natural birth, doesn't increase her risk for C-section, and doesn't mean she'll need other interventions or that her birth has become high-risk. It just means she needs to take measures to prevent transmitting the bacteria to her baby.

Yeah, but what about that IV? If a GBS-positive mother wants a low-intervention, natural labor, she can still have that. The IV site in her arm won't alter that much at all. Having an IV inserted is routine in most hospital-based labors. It's mandatory for women who want an epidural, and it provides access for an IV infusion when a woman needs rapid hydration, medications, or to be prepped for surgery. Once the IV site is established, it can be capped off and taped up so it doesn't limit a woman's mobility. She can still get into a tub, change positions, or go for a walk. She doesn't need to be continuously hooked up to tubing, a bag of solution, or an IV pole and pump unless she's actually getting medication.

Can a GBS-positive mother still have a midwife attend her birth or deliver at home or in a birth center? Sure, as long as the midwife can give her IV antibiotics during labor. If she can't do that, the mother may need to change her birth plan.

The American Pregnancy Association says that approximately one out of every 200 babies whose mothers carry GBS and are not treated with antibiotics will develop signs and symptoms of GBS disease.[2] The Centers for Disease Control says those risks drop to one baby in 4,000 when mothers are treated with antibiotics.[3] In the United States, about 1,200 babies per year become infected with GBS.

Are there natural or alternative ways to treat GBS in advance of birth? The CDC says there aren't any consistently effective ways to treat GBS and prevent transmission to babies other than IV antibiotics during labor. Some midwives and homeopaths offer garlic, acidophilus, or herb-based or other nondrug therapies and report good outcomes.

You're dilating early or not dilating yet— what now?

At some point during the last weeks of pregnancy, your provider may do a vaginal exam. She'll check whether your cervix is dilated (opening) and effaced (thinned) and whether it is soft or firm. She'll also check baby's station (location of the head in the birth canal). She'll report her findings like this: "You're closed, thick, and high," or maybe, "You're 1 centimeter, 50-percent effaced, and –2 station." Or maybe she'll say, "Whoa, you're already 4 centimeters and 100-percent effaced and this baby's head is really low." If you hear the first, you might leave your appointment thinking you're never going to dilate, labor is never going to start, and you're going to be the only woman in *Ripley's Believe It or Not* who is pregnant for the rest of her life. If you hear the last, you might think labor is imminent and you'd better put your suitcase in the car.

Here's the thing, though. The state of your cervix at one of these exams is not really an accurate estimate of when you're going to go into labor. A cervix can change super fast when it's ready. A woman who is closed, thick, and high one day can be in rockin' hard labor the next and pushing her baby out within hours. Lots of women walk around for weeks dilated 4 or 5 centimeters.

I know a few doctors who tell their 36/37-week patients that if they're not starting to dilate already, that's an indicator they may not be able to deliver vaginally. That's not true. In fact, it's nonsense. It's only an indicator that her cervix is staying closed because the uterus still has work to do to develop that baby to perfection. I know women who were told they were already starting to dilate so they might as well head to the hospital. They were told they were probably already in early labor, despite the fact that they weren't having contractions. Once they were admitted to the hospital, their doctor ruptured the water bag, hooked up the Pitocin, and added layer upon layer of unneeded interventions. It all started with a routine, late-pregnancy, let's-just-see-what's-going-on vaginal exam.

Is there any value to doing those late-pregnancy vaginal exams? Sure; in some cases they provide valuable information. But in others they provide discouragement, a false sense of urgency, and anxiety. Just because they're routine doesn't mean you have to have one. If you're just dying to know what your cervix is doing, go ahead and get the exam, but don't make any big plans based on the results. If you'd just as soon opt out, tell your provider you don't want one. If she insists, ask how the information she gathers will change your pregnancy or prenatal care. If she doesn't have a good reason or a convincing answer, and if you don't want a vaginal exam, just say "No thanks."

Your midwife says you need an obstetrician— a few reasons why you might "risk out" for low-risk/low-intervention care

You've sailed through your pregnancy without a single problem, but now your midwife says your blood sugar or blood pressure is too high and she wants you to see an obstetrician. Or maybe your baby is developing complications or your placenta isn't functioning well.

Maybe your baby is in a weird position or your placenta is covering the cervix. These are just a few common concerns a midwife might have that indicate you need a higher level of care than she feels safe providing. What do you do now? You go see an obstetrician, get an opinion, and switch gears. If your midwife feels it's not appropriate for her to take care of you, then it's not. Presumably she knows what she's doing, what her license allows her to do, and when it's best to bump someone up to an obstetrician's care. Hopefully, the OBs your midwife works with are sensitive to the goals and plans midwifery patients are hoping to achieve and will do their best to help you have the birth you want.

Of patients who choose midwives as their primary care providers during pregnancy, only a small percentage end up transferring care to an obstetrician because they've developed complications. And often when this happens the midwife remains part of the patient's care team and the doctor and midwife work together. If your midwife says you need an OB, there are a number of things you can do to make that transition as smooth as possible:

- Ask your midwife to introduce you to your new doctor.

- Ask your doctor to review your birth plan with you.

- Ask questions, and unless you're in a huge, screaming, life-threatening emergency, know that there's always enough time to get the answers you need.

- Consider hiring a doula to support you throughout labor and help you advocate for the kind of care you want.

Guide your doctor in knowing how best to take care of you. She won't know you as well as your midwife might and won't know how much you do or don't know about your specific health situation. She also won't know your learning style or how much or little information you need. Don't be intimidated by the doctor title. She is just a person you've hired to provide information, advice, and guidance.

CHAPTER 7

When the End Is in Sight

It's during the last weeks of pregnancy that the rubber meets the road. These are the hard weeks. You're totally done with the joy of pregnancy. You're so uncomfortable and your belly's so big that it takes an intervention just to roll over in bed. If you've sailed through pregnancy so far, these weeks come as a shock, as the aches and pains multiply daily. You can't see your feet, can't tie your shoes, can't stand to wear your maternity clothes one more day, and can't wait to get that baby out. That is, until you remember what it's going to take to get that baby out. Then you just feel anxious. It's the end game, and you'll be playing it for real pretty soon—but with several weeks still to go, not soon enough.

Consider this section your survival guide for how to get through the last weeks of pregnancy when you're wide open for big changes but totally vulnerable, too. As you prepare the nursery and make weekly treks to your midwife or doctor's office, you're going to need a few coping skills, from what to do when your provider throws a few curve balls into your pregnancy or birth plan to the what-if's and how-to's of induction. We'll talk about what's going on down there and what's leaking out, how to build a birth plan, and a whole lot more. Get ready to play the end game.

You know the end is in sight and all of a sudden you're freaking out— what's going on?

Your due date is coming up fast and you can finally see the light at the end of the tunnel, but instead of feeling anticipation and excitement, you're feeling anxious, sad, and afraid. That light feels like it's signaling a train speeding toward you and there's no chance you can get out of the way. Guess what? You're right on track. That train is your new life—your life as a mother—and you're right, you're going to get hit no matter what you do. The only way to get past this train is to go through labor and childbirth, meet your baby, and embrace your brand-new role in life. If that's not a great opportunity for a freak-out, then I don't know what is.

As real as pregnancy is, it's also kind of dreamy. You know you're becoming a mother, but you're not one yet (well, you are, but not tangibly). Your marriage or relationship is changing, but it's still just the two of you. You're probably still working as a nonmom, without the challenges of daycare. You're climbing up the diving board to motherhood, but the actual jump is still a ways off. And then the last month arrives and everything you've anticipated and dreamed of is becoming real. It's really about to happen. You're on the very tip of the diving board now and there's no turning back. If you're not feeling at least a little bit of fear, it's probably because either you're not acknowledging all that you're feeling or you've already had babies.

For first-time mothers, it shows good sense to experience ambivalent, even fearful, emotions at this time in your life. There aren't many bigger personal changes you'll go through. Sure, college, marriage, buying a house, your first big career, and so on are all biggies, but having a baby turns you into someone you've never been before—someone's mother. It really is a life-changer. Before kids, you're just yourself. After, you're someone's mother. Childbirth also poses a potential threat to your health and safety, no matter how healthy you are. It's potentially risky, and while your chances of coming through labor and birth safely and well are excellent, it's still a big physical hurdle, and on some level you know these things. Anxiety is to be expected.

If you're having your second child, you know what to expect from childbirth (in general; admittedly, each is different), and you've already embraced yourself as a mother. What you don't know is how on earth you're going to manage two children. You don't know how your firstborn will react to your secondborn. Will she be jealous the way you would be if your husband brought home a new wife? Will you be able to love your new baby as much as you love your first one? How do mothers chase toddlers or tame tantrums while simultaneously breastfeeding a newborn? There's a lot to think about, and even if you're pretty confident in your mothering skills, the list of unknowns is long. Anxiety is to be expected.

I'd venture to guess that if you're having your third, fourth, or ninth baby, you're probably feeling a bit more relaxed than first- or second-time mothers. You've got this. Sure, a lot of how things will proceed depends on whom you give birth to. You know each baby is different, and the exact techniques you'll use to juggle are still to be determined, but you already know you'll survive the sleepless nights, weeks of colic, and years of sibling rivalry ahead. You've already figured out the daycare, how to divide and conquer with your partner, and what married life means now that you're parents. You wouldn't go so far as to say you're totally relaxed—I mean, you still have to go through the birth process—but you know you're not facing a train wreck. Just another transformation.

How do you deal with this freak-out stage of pregnancy? Accept it as normal, even healthy. Share your feelings with the people who care about you. Talk it out, if that helps, but don't dwell on it too much. You have so many other things to think about that you really can't afford to make anxiety the main focus of your attention. Distract yourself by tidying up your work life before you head out on maternity leave. Do meditation and prenatal yoga. Go to the movies, not only to distract yourself but also because movies sans babies are a real luxury. Go out to lunch, clean your house, take long walks, make love with your partner, get massages, and redirect your focus to all the blessings and gifts that are coming your way.

I'll leave you with this: You are going to be a good mother. You will love your baby. Your partner is going to be a great parent.

Your relationship will be better than ever. Your finest hours are ahead of you, and that light at the end of the tunnel is your future self, shining a beacon of light and hope that your family will rely on. Don't worry, mama . . . you've got this.

You feel heavy, cranky, crampy, and yucky—should you ask for an induction?

I think pregnancy lasts 40 weeks because the last few weeks can be so miserable that we start to think labor is a great idea. Before that point, pregnancy is fairly tolerable (and for some women, even fun) and labor seems like something to be avoided at all costs. But virtually every one of us feels like crap during the last month we're pregnant. We ache and have cramps; we're swollen, exhausted, huge; and baby's every kick, nudge, and roll is guaranteed to hit one of our vital organs.

Over the last couple of decades many women avoided this stage altogether by asking for or agreeing to an induction. In fact, between 1990 and 2012, induction of labor rose from 9.5 to 23.3 percent of all labors.[1] Doctors didn't see any harm in recommending or agreeing to inductions for nonmedical reasons and mothers were delighted to have a few miserable days or weeks cut off the end of their pregnancies. Over time, doctors, midwives, and mothers began to realize that many of those inductions done for nonmedical indications turned into C-sections when mom's body wasn't really ready to labor and deliver. As the U.S. C-section rate climbed higher and higher, it became clearer that unnecessary inductions were doing more harm than good.

If you feel heavy, cranky, crampy, and yucky and your due date (aka the finish line) is within a week or two (or three), should you be induced? No!

Medical inductions take place in the hospital, using cervical ripening agents and medications to stimulate and regulate contractions. Inductions do have a legitimate purpose—a very specific one. They're designed to shortcut a pregnancy that's experiencing problems. For example, if a woman's blood pressure is going up, her baby isn't growing properly, her placenta is malfunctioning, or she's experiencing some other medical complication, then an induction is warranted. Sometimes the best way to protect a mother or baby's health is to serve up an eviction notice and get that kid out.

There are a few, very rare *nonmedical* reasons why an induction might be in a woman's best interest. For example, when a woman has a history of extremely fast labors and she lives 100 miles from the hospital and has a bunch of kids who need childcare, she just might need an induction to prevent her from delivering in her living room in front of her kids. Or consider another woman who has already delivered a baby vaginally and is 4 centimeters dilated; her due date is tomorrow and her husband is being deployed in a few days. These are pretty compelling situations where a nonmedical induction might be a good plan.

How about when mom is a first-timer who hasn't delivered yet but bought a too-early plane ticket so her own mother could be at her side? Nope. Not a good enough reason. How about the mother who wants her baby to be born before her doctor goes on vacation? Nope. The mother who wants to be sure her baby isn't born on a major holiday? Nope.

Inductions are way, way, way overprescribed. They're convenient, organized, and easy on the calendar, but they're also among the leading reasons why our C-section rate is so high (which is one of the leading reasons why our maternal mortality and injury rates are rising). Unless there's a *really* good reason, you don't want an induction. Inductions mess with Mother Nature's plan for when you should give birth, and Mother Nature doesn't necessarily cooperate well with people who mess with her, especially not first-time mothers.

Your body has a lot of prelabor finish work and preparation to complete before it is ready for labor. Your baby is busy, too, taking care of things like final respiratory and neural development and weight gain. There's a sort of magic (aka chemical and hormonal reactions) that happens between the baby and mom's body that sets labor in motion. When labor starts spontaneously (on its own, without induction), it has a better chance of progressing normally. Induction, on the other hand, has a fairly high failure rate, which means the baby might not descend into the birth canal well or the cervix might not dilate properly. That leads to C-sections, which leads to longer recovery times and usually to subsequent C-sections when mom gets pregnant again. It also leads to babies who aren't quite ready to be born winding up in the NICU.

Inductions of mothers who are really ready to go into labor can result in normal vaginal births (and usually do). But if your body isn't ready to get down to the business of giving birth, then you're just asking for trouble. It's far better to deal with the discomforts of late pregnancy and wait for your body to do what it was designed to do—give birth at the most optimal time for you and your baby.

What if your doctor is urging you to be induced? Ask why she thinks an induction is necessary. If her reasons aren't based on solid medical evidence, just say "No thanks." If she says it's because she's "not sure you can push out a baby that's any bigger than it is now," say, "Let's make that decision after I've pushed for a few hours." If it's because she thinks "you'll go into labor soon anyway," say, "Then let's wait for it to happen on its own." If she says it's because "I'm leaving town and I know you don't want to deliver with someone you don't know," say, "Darn, I'll miss you! But why don't you introduce me to the doctor who will be taking call for you." But if she says, "Your blood pressure's really high and I think your baby's in trouble," then by all means say, "Sign me up for that induction."

How to get the show on the road— what works and what doesn't for starting labor naturally

Most women won't need medical induction (and shouldn't want one unless they have a medical reason, as discussed earlier), but they also don't necessarily want to be pregnant forever. So what about natural techniques? You know, those time-honored methods that women have shared for generations? There are lots of myths and legends, and just as many opinions about which of these natural techniques will and won't get labor started.

If you're at or past your due date and you really can't stand being pregnant one more day, you can give these DIY, at-home tips a try. They're not guaranteed to work, but if they don't kickstart your labor, they'll at least keep you busy while you're waiting.

Before we begin, though, let me give you a heads-up. These techniques span a range from "stuff that rarely works" to things that are kind of gross to activities that may or may not be fun to things that are downright unappealing. The bottom line is, if your body isn't ready for labor, nothing you do is likely to change that. If it's teetering on the edge of labor, though, and just needs something to push it over, well then, you might get lucky.

- **Food**—Spicy food, Indian food, arugula, pizza, a big meal, Mexican food, and eggplant parmigiana are all said to induce labor. Does it work? Maybe yes, maybe no; maybe indigestion, maybe intestinal cramps—why not give it a try?

- **Castor oil**—Drinking castor oil acts as a powerful intestinal stimulant that then triggers the uterus to contract, too. Does it work? A study conducted back in 2000 divided 103 pregnant women who were between 40 and 42 weeks gestation into two groups.[2] One group of 52 women received 60 ml (about 4 tablespoons) of castor oil orally and the other (48 women) received nothing. Thirty women in the castor oil group started labor within 24 hours compared to only two in the "nothing" group. A similar study was done in 2006 with similar results: about 54 percent of women who used castor oil went into labor within 24 hours.[3] It seems to work at least half the time. However, if it does work, then in addition to being in labor and experiencing uterine contractions, you'll also experience massive intestinal cramps and possibly oily diarrhea.

- **Herbal supplements**—Evening primrose oil, black cohosh, and red raspberry leaves are the most commonly recommended herbs (by midwives and naturopaths) for starting labor. They're sometimes used in combination and sometimes alone. Their exact action isn't clear, but they may work as a cervical ripening agent (which gets the cervix ready to dilate), and they may stimulate contractions. Does it work? There aren't any clinical studies to support their effectiveness, but many midwives and women report they're safe and effective. Are they safe to use during pregnancy? There are varying opinions, probably because there aren't many studies done on their use and effects.

- **Acupuncture**—In traditional Chinese medicine, placing small sterile needles on several specific points on the body (which must be done by a trained, licensed, professional acupuncturist) is intended to stimulate the flow of energy (chi) throughout the body. When placed in certain points, this may stimulate release of prostaglandins and oxytocin, which can stimulate labor. Does it work? There aren't enough clinical studies to say for sure, but many, many women and acupuncturists claim it does. Women in many Eastern cultures use acupuncture for all kinds of medical needs, including induction of labor and pain relief, and find that it works well. There really aren't any negative side effects, so why not give this a try?

- **Nipple stimulation**—Tweaking, rolling, sucking, pumping (with a breast pump), massaging, or rubbing the nipples with a washcloth causes a natural release of oxytocin that often leads to contractions. When nipples are stimulated during pregnancy, many women notice mild contractions, but they aren't strong enough or regular enough to start labor. Does it work? When a woman is already at or past her due date, nipple stimulation may be effective for starting labor. Generally, however, it causes contractions only while the nipples are being stimulated, and they subside quickly after stimulation is discontinued. An analysis of six medical trials[4] compared results of breast stimulation with no intervention. Within 72 hours, 93 percent of women in the nipple-stimulation group were in labor compared to 62.7 percent of the no-nipple-stimulation group. This success rate may be related in part because partners often have sex after nipple stimulation, which may cause labor to start. Side note: A not-too-surprising number of partners are more than happy to give this technique a try, especially if it's followed up with sex.

- **Sex**—Not just any kind of sex. It has to include vaginal penetration that results in the man ejaculating inside the vagina. This may cause a release of prostaglandin hormones that may stimulate labor. Prostaglandins are present in both semen and cervical mucus, and they may be enough to get the ball rolling. Intercourse, like nipple stimulation, should be strictly an at-home activity. Yes, I have walked into patient rooms when couples were trying this DIY approach in the hospital. Seriously, folks—if you're in the hospital, just *don't*. Does it work? Lots of women for many generations say it does. As for official studies, research published in the journal *Obstetrics and Gynecology* says that having frequent sex close to your due date can reduce the need for induction. Another study, however, says, it doesn't work and in fact could delay labor. Another study says sex alone won't do it, but nipple stimulation during sex might. As long as you're past your due date and have no medical reasons why you shouldn't have sex, having sex to start labor is certainly worth a try.

How to keep from losing your mind while you wait for labor to start

Somewhere around week 38, some women convince themselves the baby's going to be born any minute. (The rest feel like they'll be pregnant forever.) It doesn't matter that their due date isn't for two more weeks or that many babies need an extra week or two in the oven beyond their due date to bake to perfection. These moms can't imagine being any more uncomfortable, any bigger, or any more "due" than they already are; therefore, they become certain that labor's going to start any minute. Except that it usually doesn't. Instead, most pregnancies drag on the full-allotted time period. This makes mothers nutty, which is why you need an action plan for how to avoid losing your mind while you wait for labor to start.

It's during these last few weeks that many mothers become susceptible to their doctors' subtle suggestions. Doctors know you're freaking miserable and might say something like, "You know . . . we could just go ahead and break your water or start a little Pitocin and you could have this baby today." Many well-intentioned mothers take the bait and decide to just go for it. What could it hurt? You're almost due, right? Yeah, well, maybe so and maybe no. Unless you have a medical reason, don't go for an induction. (For more on inductions, see page 96.)

The weeks drag on even more slowly if your provider suggests you'll deliver sooner than later, like when your midwife says, "You're already 2 centimeters dilated. I think you'll have your baby this weekend." Except the weekend comes and goes and there you are, still pregnant. That's why it's not always such a great idea to have that end-of-pregnancy vaginal exam. If it doesn't make a difference, why torture yourself?

What can you do to ride out the last few weeks (or more) without totally losing your mind or succumbing to unnecessary medical interventions? It's all about distraction, baby: movies, books, walks, chores, dinners out, exercise, sleep, errands—whatever it takes to pass the time. Play mental games with yourself that you're guaranteed to win. "If I'm still not in labor by the end of the day, I'll treat myself to a new pair of socks." Or pretend your due date is two weeks later than it really is. That way you won't feel so frantic when you're looking at your real due date in the rearview mirror.

One woman I know asked each of her friends to organize a "save the day" game plan that covered the two weeks before her due date and a week after. Her friends divided up the calendar and planned a day of company, gentle activities, little outings, and small presents all designed to make each day she didn't go into labor a special one.

Another woman knew her family would start pestering her with "Are you in labor?" phone calls as soon as her due date was a month away. So she bent the truth and said her due date was a week later than it was. Yeah, she felt bad about lying, but she bought herself an extra week of peace.

Personally, I approached my due date with baby number two from the opposite end of the spectrum. My due date coincided with the day I was scheduled to take final exams for nursing school. My first baby had been two weeks late, so I counted on this one being tardy, too. If she came early, I wouldn't be able to take final exams and I'd have to repeat the semester (they were real hard-asses at my school). My baby must have known this was serious, because she not only let me take finals on my due date but also let me walk across the graduation stage and receive my diploma three days later and tacked on an extra four-day break after graduation before making her appearance.

Remember, your due date is just an *estimation* of when you'll go into labor. Try not to take it too seriously. Babies know better than almost anyone else when it's the right day to be born. Just stay busy, get some rest, and know that nobody is pregnant forever.

You're overdue (or are you?)— what should you do?

We've talked a lot in this section about managing expectations around your due date, avoiding inductions, how to get labor started naturally, and the value of letting labor start when baby is darn good and ready. But going past your due date makes doctors and some midwives really nervous. Once that 40-week mile-marker is within sight, some doctors start putting on the pressure. They drop worry bombs like, "You know the placenta won't work forever, right?" or "That baby's sure getting big. I'm not sure you can push it out." Or they simply go all father or mother figure on you: "I'm not going to *let you* go past your due date." But again, the due date is just an estimate, not a precise date when baby must be born or else. In most cases, nothing bad happens if the timer goes off and labor hasn't started.

What about the placenta? It's true that after a certain point, usually after 42 weeks, the placenta can become too old to function properly. It's designed to be a temporary body organ, and in most pregnancies, birth happens before the placenta reaches its "best used by" date. If the placenta malfunctions before birth, it can seriously impact baby's health by decreasing circulation, oxygenation, and waste management in the uterus. The placenta may age more rapidly in mothers with diabetes or those who smoke, take drugs, or have other health conditions. If a placenta is compromised by calcification or because it's positioned in a weird way in the uterus, this can also cause it to fail sooner rather than later. A normal, healthy placenta, however, will last for the duration, and if you're not past 42 weeks, there's very little reason to worry about it.

How can you tell if the placenta is still working? If the baby is moving normally, chances are good the placenta is fine. If not, let your doctor know, and she can do a nonstress test to determine fetal well-being.

What about the baby getting too big? Your body was designed to deliver a normal-size baby. What's normal for one woman is a matter of genetics, health, and both her size and the baby's father's size. Our bodies are designed to birth the babies we produce, and in most cases there is no weight limit (within reason). Some women have a particularly narrow pelvis that won't allow for a vaginal birth, but this is rare. That's why it's best to give labor a try, even when a big baby is suspected. We really don't know how big a baby is going to be before she's born. Ultrasounds are notoriously inaccurate at predicting an exact weight, and so is the old-school hands-on-the-belly method. Both techniques might provide an estimate, but they can't say for sure that "this baby is too big to be born vaginally." When labor is allowed to start on its own and proceed without too much intervention and without a stopwatch, most women are able to deliver whatever size baby they have produced.

"Why won't my doctor 'let me' go past my due date?" That's a classic control issue, probably based on his fear that something might go wrong. He may have been trained that anything past 40 weeks is abnormal (it's not) or that the placenta will short-circuit at any moment (it probably won't), or perhaps he doesn't know how to maneuver larger babies (he *should* know) or he doesn't want the inconvenience of not knowing when you're going to deliver (too bad—not your problem). This approach, when doctors say they won't "let" their patients do something, really bugs me. Doctors are not in charge of their patients. Mothers are not children who need to be given permission or told what to do. Mothers are adults in charge of their own bodies, and they pay their doctors for advice and information. What they do with that information is up to them.

If you're overdue and you're not experiencing any medical complications, try not to worry. Your body and your baby will choose the right birthday. If your doctor is pressuring you, ask what he's so worried about. If all he has are "what if" scenarios that have nothing to do with you and your individual pregnancy, feel free to give him the same advice: "Try not to worry. My baby and my body will choose the best birthday."

It won't hurt to try some of the things we outlined earlier in this book (page 98) for getting the show on the road. It probably also won't hurt to just chill out and know it's going to happen soon. If you've gone past 42 weeks, though, we're talking about increased risk of problems. It's quite possible you're not as far along as you think, but it's also possible you'll need more advanced monitoring. This is what nonstress tests and biophysical profiles are for—to determine which babies and placentas are still fine right where they are and which babies need to be born. If at any point you feel "weird" or your baby isn't moving properly, tell your doctor you're worried, and let her outline next steps.

CHAPTER 8

Are You in Labor?

You're having contractions, leaking some fluid, and you're pretty sure the big day is finally here! But are you really, truly in honest-to-god labor? Maybe. Unless you've had a baby before, it can be really hard to tell. Let's talk it through and set some guidelines for how to know when you are or aren't in labor.

You're leaking fluid—did your water break or did you wet your pants?

Once past their own toddler years, few women need to worry about wetting their pants in public. All that changes during pregnancy. In fact, there's a small but distinct possibility that you really might be out at the market or in the theater when all of a sudden the flood happens (aka, your water breaks). That's called "spontaneous rupture of membranes" or SROM. There you'll be in all your glorious wetness with a puddle at your feet and a baby on the way—just like in the movies. That is, unless you've simply peed your pants. What? You think that won't happen to you? Guess again. On the maternity unit, we see women in all stages of dampness, and more often than not, it's *not* because their water has broken.

Here's what happens: A mother feels a sudden gush of fluid and thinks, *This is it!* She calls her provider and says, "I think my water broke," and her doc or midwife says, "Go to the hospital and we'll check that out." She's told to wear a pad to collect any further leakage, but hopefully she's advised to *not* alert her family and labor support crew until it's absolutely certain her water broke.

When she arrives on the unit, her nurse will ask her to undress and to leave her pad and/or wet clothing in the bathroom. Mom will get into bed, where a big blue waterproof paper-lined pad placed underneath her butt will collect any fluid she's continuing to leak. The nurse will place fetal heart and contraction monitoring equipment on mom's belly and then ask a whole lot of really personal questions. That's because determining what caused mom's wet underwear isn't as clear-cut as most women think. The questions will go something like this:

- What happened when your underwear got wet?

- Was it a big gush or a trickle?

- Did fluid continue to leak out or was it a onetime thing?

- Were you able to make the leakage stop?

- Was there any color or smell to the fluid?

- When was the last time you had sex?

- Are you having any cramps or contractions?

- Is there any spotting or bleeding?

Your answers help guide the nurse to determine what exactly came out. You're probably wondering about that sex question, right? I can't tell you how many times (lots of times, seriously, lots and lots) the answer was, "About an hour ago, and that's when something started leaking out." Yep, that happens. If that's the case, we go through a few diagnostic formalities to determine that the "something" is actually semen, and we send the embarrassed mom home with reassurance and a wee bit of education.

If she answers yes to the questions about color, smell, and ability to control the leak, we're probably looking at urine, not amniotic fluid. The odor of amniotic fluid reminds some people of salt water or the ocean, but it does *not* smell like urine. Amniotic fluid is mostly clear; there may be white flecks in it or small streaks of blood, but it isn't supposed to be yellow (if it is, that signals infection or the presence of meconium—baby poop). Cramping and contractions? A constant leakage or a big gush? Now it's starting to sound like amniotic fluid.

Next, using mom's pad, clothing, the pad under her tush, and/or the fluid collecting on the outside of her vagina, the nurse will use Nitrazine paper, a yellow test strip that turns blue in the presence of amniotic fluid. It also sometimes turns blue in the presence of mucus, blood, and other fluids, so it's not an exact diagnostic tool, but it gives a pretty clear indication. If there's not much fluid present and nothing makes the test strip turn blue, our hunches are that it's urine, semen, or just a lot of vaginal discharge. We may do a sterile speculum exam. We'll insert the speculum, shine a light into the far end of the vagina, and look for fluid pooling near the cervix. We'll test that fluid with Nitrazine paper and use a large sterile swab to absorb whatever we see in the vagina or on the speculum. We'll wipe the swab across microscope slides, let it dry, and then look at the slides under a microscope. Amniotic fluid dries into distinct salt crystals that look like fern fronds. They're quite beautiful and very distinct. If we see ferning, we know the woman's water has broken and her labor is on the way.

What if the Nitrazine paper is negative (doesn't turn blue) and there's no ferning? Then mom joins the legions of other mothers who are probably leaking urine. As embarrassing as that sounds, it's incredibly common. As baby's head presses on the bladder, mom can hold less and less fluid. Some of it is bound to leak out without her being aware of it, especially if she makes sudden movements, waits too long to pee, sneezes, coughs, exercises, or for no reason at all. It happens all the time. It happened to me when I was pregnant, and I'd wager that it happened to most of the nurses I've worked with when they were pregnant.

Only about 10 to 20 percent of women have their water break before labor starts. When this does happen, contractions generally begin within the next 24 hours. If SROM happens several weeks before the baby is full term, the doctor might try to stall labor by using medications and bed rest (usually in the hospital) to buy baby more time in the uterus. If it happens after 35 weeks, chances are good that even if baby is born early, he will be perfectly fine.

If you leak fluid, should you assume you're in the 10 to 20 percent with SROM or the 80 to 90 percent who are leaking something else? You shouldn't make any assumptions at all. Call your provider and let her guide you. Many women think it's a bad thing to go into the maternity unit for evaluation unless you're absolutely in labor. That's not true. In fact, most maternity units have a couple of rooms (or even a whole area) and nurses staffed specifically for these kinds of evaluations. They're important, common, and 100-percent normal. If you need to be checked out, so be it. Don't worry about being judged, sent home, or embarrassed. You won't be judged, you may be sent home, but honey, we've seen it all, and nothing you have to show us will be any different from what a dozen other women have shown us that week. You're among friends. You're with women who know. Let us take care of you.

You lost your mucous plug or see a little bleeding—are you going into labor?

All hail the mucous plug. It's the stuff that dreams are made of for many women who believe that once that glob comes out, labor is mere hours away. They welcome it like it's their beloved returning from a long trip or a sign from the universe that foretells great riches. Alas, it's just a glob of mucus, and many women lose it days or weeks before labor starts. Many women never even notice when it comes out.

I remember expecting that the mucous plug would come out like a cork. I literally thought of it as a plug, and when instead it appeared in chunks and drips and like snot, I was really disappointed (and a little grossed out). For some women it does pop out in one piece, but for most, it's more like an ongoing process of heavy discharge. It might be creamy, brown, blood tinged, or yellowish. It might be thick or liquid, or so nondescript that it blends in with all the other discharge from the vagina.

Does it signal the beginning of the end? Well, yes, sort of, as long as you think of "the end" as some distant point remotely near your due date, give or take a week or so. I think it's better to view losing your mucous plug as just one more weird thing that happens during the last month. It doesn't mean that labor is imminent. It also doesn't mean you need to collect it on a piece of tissue paper and bring it to your doctor or the hospital for evaluation. You really don't. It's just mucus.

How about "bloody show"? This is very light bleeding or spotting, often mixed with discharge or mucus. It should not fill up a pad. If your due date is soon, bloody show might indicate labor is imminent—or it might not. Bloody show is an indication that your cervix is starting to change. It may be effacing (thinning out), softening, and dilating, and in the process, tiny blood vessels break or leak fluid. It might mean you're in the early stages of labor, but it might also happen a week or so before you go into labor. It might happen in fits and spurts, meaning your sensitive cervix spots a little any time it does a little work. You might have some show one day and then nothing for a week, have a little more, then nothing again for a while.

Any amount of bleeding should be mentioned to your provider, but in most cases it's OK to start with a phone call, not a trip to the hospital.

How will you know if it's bloody show or something more serious? Unless you've experienced bloody show before, you might not know, so let your midwife or doc guide you. Put on a pad to protect your clothing, and if that pad fills up quickly, that's not "show." If the bleeding is heavy, especially if it's associated with abdominal pain or lack of fetal movement, that could be serious. Heavy bleeding can indicate the placenta is separating from the uterus early or that it's covering the cervix—both are serious and need immediate medical attention. Call your provider or the hospital, and if they tell you to go in for evaluation, go.

How to tell when you're really, truly, honest-to-god in labor

When I was pregnant with my first baby, I'd already been working in women's health for almost ten years. I'd been a medical assistant for a few obstetricians, been present at a few labors, seen a couple of babies born, taken Lamaze classes, and I had sisters with babies, so basically that made me an expert on what it meant to be "in labor." Right?

There I was, ten days overdue and having regular contractions. My belly was getting tight at regular intervals, and most of these contractions hurt (more or less). I'd lost my mucous plug and was having some bloody show. I was edgy and cranky as hell and pretty darn sure I was in labor. My husband dutifully timed and recorded my contractions all night long, and when, in the morning, I felt sure I was on my way, we drove to my OB's office for a labor check. He examined my cervix and told me as kindly as possible that I was only a fingertip dilated, but he was certain labor would start within a few days.

"A few days? What the hell have I been doing all this time if that wasn't labor?"

I'd been experiencing what we call prelabor (the medical term is prodromal labor). That's the disorganized, time-consuming, annoying, and exhausting preamble to real labor.

It's not "false labor." These contractions are performing important functions. They're getting baby into a good birthing position and as low in the pelvis as possible without pulling out the big guns (aka real, true labor contractions). They're getting the cervix ripe and ready by helping it soften, thin out, and move from a posterior position (tucked way up at the top of the vagina) to an anterior position (lower in the vagina, with the cervical os/opening toward the front). It's unfortunate that dilation gets all the attention in the labor show, but this effacement and ripening must happen before the cervix can really get down to the business of dilating.

I asked my doctor how I would know when I was really in labor, and he said, "Oh, you'll know. Believe me, you'll know." Well, of course, he was spot-on correct. The irritating pattern of on-again, off-again contractions continued for another day before we turned a great big corner. Then my contractions became regular and much stronger, and we weren't messing around anymore.

Many labors (especially those of first-timers) start with prodromal labor. How will you know when you're really in labor? Well, I hate to make this sound too ominous, but pain is a big indicator. Real labor contractions don't just feel like bad menstrual cramps. They may start out that way, but they move on and beyond to something very different and, for most women, a lot worse than bad cramps. Your back and legs may also hurt during contractions and you may experience some intestinal action (aka diarrhea). Your contractions will become regular and progressively closer together. Eventually you'll have a contraction every two to three minutes, and they'll each last a minute or so. That may mean you get only a minute off between contractions.

Here are some hints that you're not yet in labor:

- You're having regular contractions but you don't really have to break your stride when you're having one.

- You can still talk through contractions, breathe normally, make sandwiches, and carry on about your business.

- Your contractions are regular and strong until you climb into the tub, lie down, or go for a walk, at which point they space apart.

- Some contractions are painful, but others aren't.

For those who say contractions (or surges) aren't painful, just intense—feel free to substitute the word "intense" wherever you like. The principle is the same—if your surges aren't regular and increasingly intense and powerful, it's not labor.

If you have to catch your breath and stop talking or doing anything else in order to cope with your contraction, now you're onto something. If they go from ten to seven to five to three minutes apart and stay that close together, it's starting to look like labor. If your contractions are no more than five minutes apart and getting stronger no matter what you do (bathe, rock, walk, sleep), you're probably in labor. If you're contracting away and your water breaks—yes, that's probably labor.

If your water breaks and you're not contracting yet, however, you're not actually in labor, though you're definitely on your way. Depending on your midwife/doctor's preferences, the color of the fluid, your baby's position and activity level, and whether or not you're running a fever, you may be advised to go to the hospital right away or, ideally, told to stay at home until you're having regular contractions and are in honest-to-goodness labor. Most doctors want you to be in labor within 24 hours of rupturing your membranes because they're worried about infection setting in. If nobody checks your cervix, though (and you don't put anything else in your vagina), your chances of becoming infected are pretty low.

Real labor consists of strong, regular contractions that cause progressive cervical change. When you go to the hospital, if your water has not broken, you'll probably have a cervical exam. If you're contracting up a storm but your cervix isn't changing, you're not in active labor yet. If your cervix isn't dilated very far or changing, you may even be sent home. Don't worry about that. Nobody will judge you. We'll think you were smart to come in and get checked.

If your prelabor contractions have been going on for a ridiculously long time and you're exhausted and can't sleep, you may be offered some narcotic medication to provide "therapeutic rest." At my hospital we gave patients who are having disorganized contractions a big ol' shot of morphine to relieve the pain and put a stop to contractions long enough that the patient could grab some sleep. Very often, when she woke up she'd be in active labor.

We used to identify the stages of labor based on how far you were dilated, like this:

1–3 centimeters: early labor

4–7 centimeters: active labor

8–10 centimeters: transition

Now, many midwives, doctors, and birth experts say we shouldn't call it "active labor" before 6 centimeters. I'm not sure there's an exact centimeter that defines when you're "active" and when you're "early." I like a more common sense definition: you're contracting, they're getting stronger and closer together, and your cervix is definitely changing. That's labor. And honey, there won't be any doubt in your mind about whether or not it's really, truly, honest-to-god labor. You'll know.

Water management—what to do if your water bag breaks in public and what to expect when it breaks during labor

How many TV and movie labors start with mom's water breaking in a public place? Lots and lots. How many start that way in real life? Not that many. In fact, only about 15 percent of labors start with spontaneous rupture of membranes (SROM—official medical lingo for water breaking), but the risk of its happening in public keeps 100 percent of women on their toes, certain it will happen to them.

With each pregnancy, I was sure my water would break while I was at the store, at my kids' schools or, my worst fear, when I was walking across the stage, graduating from nursing school.

When graduation day arrived and I was still pregnant, I switched my worry from *what if I don't graduate* to the next logical subject: *What if my water breaks while I'm on stage?* Never mind that I'd be on stage getting my diploma for approximately 15 seconds. No amount of logic could convince me it would happen any other way. There I'd be, shaking our principal's hand when—gush, splash!—my water would break and flood the stage. Then, of course, I'd immediately be overcome with contractions (just like on TV) and all the brand-new nurses graduating with me would rush to my side and deliver my baby right there on stage. No matter that I already had one baby or that I had worked in labor and delivery and knew full well birth didn't happen that way. Logic be damned—being overdue messed with my mind, and hormones fueled my imagination. I prepared for the dam breaking, subsequent flood and onstage delivery by stockpiling giant feminine hygiene pads. I wore two under my spiffy white maternity nursing uniform. Just to give you the full visual, this was back in the day when nursing students had to wear nursing hats that made us look like the Flying Nun.

So, did it happen? Did I create a huge puddle right there in front of several hundred of my co-graduates' families? Of course not. My water broke several days later during labor, just as it does for most women.

Even though it's not likely you'll wet yourself in public, it's good to have an action plan in place, just in case. You can, of course, start wearing the huge pads when you're nearing your due date, but they're not that comfortable. A more practical approach is to stash pads and a change of clothing in a tote bag, along with a big towel. Stow it in your car and consider that your insurance policy. Seriously, what else can you do? If it breaks, it breaks, and most people will dodge out of the way of the oncoming fluid.

The amniotic membrane doesn't always break like someone took a knife to a water balloon. Instead, it's often more like somebody poked a hole in it with a pin, causing it to drip, squirt, and leak in dribs and drabs that are a bit more manageable in public places.

What does it feel like when your water breaks? If it happens on its own (SROM) you might not feel a thing other than sudden wetness. Many women feel, hear, or somehow sense the moment it happens, though they can't exactly say what they felt or heard. There's a knowing moment that's followed by wet underwear or a puddle in the bed or a trickle running down a leg. When my water finally broke with my "graduation baby," I was in labor, sitting on the toilet. I was 3 centimeters dilated, and my contractions were coming hard and fast. I felt a pop and heard the fluid trickle into the toilet. I knew I wasn't peeing because I couldn't control the flow. When it continued to leak out after I got off the toilet, my midwife checked the fluid with Nitrazine paper (see page 109), and sure enough, my water had broken. My daughter was born about 45 minutes later.

If your water is broken by your midwife or doctor (a procedure called artificial rupture of membranes or AROM, often done to start or speed up labor), you might not feel anything in particular other than a vaginal exam. Your provider will probably use a flat plastic instrument with a curved end that looks like a crochet hook. She'll insert it through your cervix and hook it into your amniotic membrane. We sometimes call that "snagging your bag," because that's what she's doing. The next thing you'll feel is wet, wet, wet. You'll have a pile of towels and paper-plastic pads under you to catch the flood, and you'll be given the biggest pads you've ever seen to stuff into your underwear.

Another technique for snagging your bag is to use a fetal scalp electrode (FSE), which is a tube (it looks like a long drinking straw) that contains an electronic monitoring lead with a small wire that's intended to attach to the outermost layer of skin on a baby's head. FSE is usually used to directly monitor baby's heartbeat (rather than using an external monitor on mom's belly), but the wire is also an effective tool for AROM. Once your bag is broken, you'll feel a drip, leak, trickle, or gush.

Amniotic fluid is usually clear and sometimes has white flecks in it. It smells like seawater or like clean salt water. It should not smell foul, sweet, or nasty. If it does, you may have an infection. If the fluid is brown, green, or yellow or has black flecks in it, your baby may have taken a poop in your amniotic fluid; that's called meconium. We'll talk more about meconium on page 151.

CHAPTER 9

At the Hospital

It's go time, the big day, your birth *day.* This section covers all the need-to-know items you'll deal with during labor and birth, from who works on the maternity unit to what your nurse and midwife really think about your bikini line. Buckle your seatbelts and let's get going. You're having your baby.

Who works on the maternity unit? From nurses to lab techs—all the people who might take care of you and your baby

If you're delivering your baby in a hospital maternity unit, know this: It takes a village to birth a baby—a village of health care workers and support staff whose individual jobs are interconnected to provide comprehensive patient care and support the hospital's administrative and technical needs. While you won't meet all of these people during your hospital stay, you'll definitely interact with quite a few. Who are the people in your hospital's village?

Doctors:

- **Obstetricians (OB-GYNs)** generally see patients in their offices for prenatal care and in hospitals when their patients are ready to deliver or have a C-section. The doctor who takes care of you in the hospital might be the same one you've seen throughout your pregnancy or might be one of her partners. OBs aren't on call and available every day or night of the week to deliver their own patients. Instead, they rotate call shifts with other OBs so they can get some sleep and have a life.

- **Hospitalists (aka laborists)** are doctors that work on some maternity units. Their job is to take care of women in labor while they're admitted to the hospital. They don't do prenatal care, so you may not have met your hospitalist prior to delivery. They are responsible for supervising labors, delivering babies, managing postpartum issues, doing C-sections, and taking care of triage patients who come in for reasons other than labor and delivery. The advantage of having a hospitalist is that he's focused exclusively on what's happening in the hospital and therefore not distracted by office patients or patients on other units. He also may not be as eager to implement interventions meant to speed labor along, because he's not in a hurry. He's there for the whole shift. He has a specific work schedule, so he won't have been awake for days on end managing patients in the office and in the hospital. Hospitalists often do fewer C-sections because they're located on the maternity unit (not dashing back and forth from home to office to hospital, like most OBs) and more able to take a wait-and-see approach. What's the disadvantage? Because you probably haven't met this doctor before, you won't know his style or personality or how he practices. He may also be juggling several labor patients at once, so he may be distracted and not fully focused on you.

- **Perinatologists** are obstetricians who specialize in the care of fetuses and complicated, high-risk pregnancies. Perinatology is also known as maternal-fetal medicine. They're the docs who work with diabetic patients, manage multiple pregnancies (twins, triplets), and do fetal surgery, amniocentesis, and chorionic villus sampling.

- **Neonatologists** are pediatricians who specialize in the care of newborns and preemies. Their domain is the NICU.

- **Pediatricians** take care of normal newborns. It's unlikely you'll need a pediatrician at your delivery, but she may be called in if there's a complication or if you're having twins or triplets. She'll also come to examine your baby before you're discharged to go home.

- **Family practice doctors** sometimes deliver babies and take care of postpartum mothers as well as newborns. They don't do C-sections, though, or take care of high-risk mothers.

- **Other physician specialists**—Some mothers need a lot more care than others. They may need endocrinologists, hematologists, immunologists, oncologists, psychiatrists, gastroenterologists, or other specialists. These doctors don't usually hang out on the maternity unit, but they come when they're called for patients who need them.

- **Anesthesiologists** provide pain management during surgeries and administer epidurals. They also sometimes provide respiratory support for babies who need special care or mothers who are having a crisis.

Midwives: Almost all the midwives who work in hospitals are certified nurse midwives, though in some states certified midwives (who have a different educational path) also have hospital privileges. They do almost everything OBs do except for C-sections and management of high-risk patients.

Nurses: These ladies (and a few men, but on maternity units they're mostly women) totally run the maternity ward. Most are registered nurses (RNs, with a two-year nursing education in addition to other college), but some may be licensed professional nurses (LPNs, with one year of nursing education). All have specialized training in obstetrics, mother-baby care, labor and delivery, and/or nursery/NICU care.

- **Postpartum nurses** take care of mothers after they deliver.

- **Labor and delivery nurses** take care of women before and during labor and during their births or C-sections and recovery period. They may also do postpartum care.

- **Certified nurse anesthetists** are advanced-practice nurses with a master's level education in anesthesia. They do pain management during surgeries and administer epidurals. They are also specialists in managing airways and providing respiratory support.

- **Nursery nurses** take care of newborn babies. **NICU nurses** take care of premature or sick babies.

- **Charge nurses** decide which nurses will take care of which patients. They manage the flow of patients on the unit and help facilitate procedures, surgeries, and staffing issues.

- The **nurse manager** is in charge of the entire unit. She makes administrative decisions, does hiring and firing, and manages the budgets, staffing, standards, training, and so on.

Technicians and therapists have varying levels of education and training and specialize in providing specific services:

- **Surgical techs** are responsible for setting up surgical equipment and preparing operating rooms (ORs) for surgery, assisting in surgeries by handing equipment to surgeons, and performing other OR-related duties.

- **Respiratory therapists** care for patients who have trouble breathing. They set up oxygen tents and ventilators, among other duties.

- **IV techs or IV nurses** are the experts at starting IVs. In some maternity units, labor nurses start most of the IVs, and IV specialists are called in only for patients whose veins are difficult to access. In other facilities, IV techs or IV nurses start all IVs.

- **Auditory techs** perform hearing screening tests on newborns.

- **Lab technicians/phlebotomists** draw blood and collect other lab specimens.

Support staff:

- **Unit secretaries** and **ward clerks** perform scheduling, phone, and organization/administration functions that help nurses and physicians do their jobs. They're usually located at the front desk or nurses' station—and as far as nurses are concerned, they run the world we work in.

- **Food service staffers** will bring your meals and snacks.
- **Cleaning crew members** make sure your room is spotless when you're admitted and come in daily (or more often) to keep it tidy.
- **Admissions office staff** may come by to get signatures on consents and to get insurance information.
- **Chaplains** are available for blessings, prayers, and spiritual support as needed.
- **Social workers** assist patients with emotional, physical, social, occupational, and housing needs and other special circumstances.

This is by no means a comprehensive list of people who work in hospitals, but it will help you understand what all those people in your maternity unit are doing. If you feel like your room has a revolving door, talk to your nurse or the charge nurse about traffic control or ask them to coordinate their care to minimize interruptions.

Hygiene and grooming for labor— what matters, what totally doesn't?

There aren't many times in our lives when we know we'll be pantsless in front of strangers. Oh sure, there was college and possibly a few boozy nights, but once we're beyond all that, the opportunities are generally rare. When having the baby is on the horizon, though, we know that's part of the deal. In fact, no matter how careful your nurses are to guard your privacy and modesty (and they'll do their best, I promise), it's almost guaranteed you're going to be in some level of undress in front of your nurse, midwife, doctor, and, if you have a labor entourage, your friends and family.

Some women go to a lot of trouble to tidy up their lady bits in addition to getting a pedicure and manicure, shaving their legs and armpits, and getting their makeup done and hair fixed in a perfect "in labor" style. How much of that is necessary? None of it. Your nurses aren't going to mind one bit if your toes aren't done and your legs are hairy. We don't care if you have a bikini wax, and shaving your pubic hair is

100 percent unnecessary (we no longer do that as a routine part of birth). We think wearing a lot of makeup is a waste of time, especially since you may be spending some time in a tub or shower as a means of relieving labor pain. And that "in labor" hairstyle? Seriously? How good is that going to look after 12 hours (more or less) of contractions, pushing, and sweat?

The pedicure is always a nice touch, but only because it shows that you (or someone you love) pampered yourself a bit, but other than that, none of this grooming is anything any of the people taking care of you will care about one bit. Doctors, nurses, and midwives take care of women from all walks of life, all cultures, all socioeconomic statuses and age groups. Shaving, grooming, and makeup practices vary a lot across different cultures, and we're totally respectful of that. We also know how hard it is for most pregnant women to reach their feet, legs, and nether regions during the last month, so we don't judge. Most women come in to labor with stubble and chipped polish. Heck, it's hard enough to put on your socks and tie your shoes. Shaving and polishing are darn near impossible.

How about jewelry? Leave as much as possible at home. Rings are fine, as are earrings, but if you have to go into surgery, you're very likely going to have to take them off. Wedding rings, permanent bracelets, and other nonremovable jewelry are fine, and if there are concerns about them reacting with equipment in the OR, the jewelry will be covered and taped. If you have genital piercings (yeah, that's a thing), you should remove those ornaments before you give birth. Pierced belly button? It's not absolutely necessary to take that out, unless you're having a C-section. How about nipple piercings? Take them out. Not only will they interfere with breastfeeding, but if you need emergency surgery, they might get in the way of wires, cardiac sensors, and cautery equipment.

Do we care whether you wear your own clothes? No, not really. As long as you're comfortable and your clothes are clean, you can wear what you want, but remember this: Labor and birth are a messy business, and the advantages of wearing a hospital gown are that it provides easy access and we'll do the laundry. If you wear your own gown, make sure it doesn't get mixed in with hospital laundry or you'll never see it again.

Do we care if you prefer to be totally naked? No. We understand that you're working hard and labor is hot and sweaty. If you're more comfortable in your birthday suit, that's fine. In fact, the only thing we (your nurses and care providers) ask of you is this: "If you're not in too big a hurry and if you can possibly manage it, can you please take a nice soapy shower before you come in to labor and delivery?" If the baby's on her way, though, or you don't have access to a shower or tub, don't worry about it. Seriously. Don't worry about it. Oh, and just one more thing: While we're OK with mom being naked, we're not OK with dad or other labor supporters stripping down. Seriously, guys: she can—you can't. Thanks for keeping it PG-13.

Shaving, enemas, episiotomies, and other old-school routines

So many birth plans include these mandates: No shaving, enema, or episiotomy. The mothers who include this trio often get this information from old books or Internet sites that make it sound like they're part of the routine for every birth. For the most part, they're not. These are such old-school procedures, I'm surprised they're in the books anymore. Despite the fact that these haven't been part of the routine in decades, they live on in the lore of U.S. childbirth, freaking out generations of mothers who think we're going to shave them, cut them, and make them poop. We're not. You can relax on this. That is, unless you *do* have a doctor who is practicing like it's still the 1960s. In which case, you're smart to include these items on your birth plan. Smarter still to find a doctor who's up on the new standards of care.

The shaving thing

It used to be, way back when (not while I've been a nurse, and that's been a really long time), every woman admitted for labor had her perineum shaved, probably with an old-fashioned safety razor. The thought was that it made things cleaner and easier to see, and since she was probably also going to get an episiotomy, a hair-free perineum would be easier to stitch back up. We gave up routine shaving so long ago that even nurses as old as me have never done it. Actually, that's not true; I trimmed one woman, but that was because she had so much pubic hair (like nothing I've ever seen before or since) that her baby got caught. As her baby was trying to push his way out of the vagina, he got snagged in her hair, and it was pulling on her in such an uncomfortable way that she asked me to get some scissors and cut it. I did, and once we got rid of the tangles, the baby practically fell out. No lie.

If a woman needs a C-section, we may use clippers to get rid of some of the hair at her bikini line. We don't shave off everything, but we do remove anything that covers the area of incision. That's so doctors can see where to make the incision and avoid stitching pubic hair into the cut when they're closing it back up.

Should you shave yourself? Don't bother. Lots of women come in having shaved because they think we're going to do it anyway. We're not. Some women prefer being hair-free. That's fine, but don't go to any trouble on our account. We seriously don't care how much hair you have down there.

What about the enema?

That used to be de rigueur back in the olden days, too. Since pooping during birth is super common, women were routinely given enemas during labor so they wouldn't poop when they were pushing. An enema involves inserting a tube into the rectum and flushing water and soap solution through the tube into the intestines. The water and soap irritate the bowel, which causes you to poop.

If you've ever had an enema, you know it's not comfortable. It can cause intestinal cramping like nobody's business. It also makes you feel out of control, which technically you are. Many mothers get diarrhea during labor anyway (nature's way of cleaning house), and adding an enema into the mix is pure misery. We don't do it anymore unless a particular mother asks for one or unless a midwife wants to use an enema to stimulate labor (the cramps that cause the intestines to empty also sometimes make the uterus contract).

If you don't have an enema, will you poop when you have your baby? You might. It's no big deal to those of us taking care of you, though we know it's a big deal to you. We'll keep you clean and discreet, and hopefully you'll never realize you did it. Seriously—it's no big deal.

Now, about those episiotomies

Back in the day, almost every mother received an episiotomy, which is an incision made from the lower end of the vaginal opening into the perineum. It's supposed to create room for the baby's head to get through and was thought to be easier to repair than a tear. The thing is, though, not every woman tears during birth (especially if she's given time to stretch naturally) and it turns out tears are just as easy to repair as incisions. So why cut every woman when only some will tear? Eventually, most doctors agreed that didn't make sense, and they quit doing episiotomies on every mother.

Sometimes, though, an episiotomy is necessary. About 12 percent of deliveries involve an episiotomy. If baby needs to be delivered faster than mom can stretch (for instance, if the baby's in some kind of trouble), or if forceps or a vacuum extractor is needed to facilitate a vaginal delivery, then an episiotomy can be a lifesaver. Once they're repaired, most heal well. We talk more about episiotomies in "Lacerations 101" on page 157.

What are some other misconceptions women hear about labor? There are lots. Some are cultural, some are based on ignorance, and an awful lot are urban myth. That's why it's important to get a top-notch prenatal education—to know fact from fiction.

Can you eat when you're in labor?

If it were up to me, I'd say "yes" every time. Hunger is a pretty good sign that your body wants calories. Since labor is a lot of physical work, it makes sense that you might want something to eat at some point. It's not up to me, though, so here's the scoop on eating while in labor: it depends on whom you ask and where you deliver.

If you deliver at home with a midwife, you'll be encouraged to eat and drink whatever and whenever you want. You may be ravenous and want to eat three square meals while you're laboring, or you may not have much of an appetite. It's up to you: feel free to nibble or not. Some women feel sick to their stomach during labor and aren't into eating. Let your body be your guide.

If you're at a birth center, chances are good you'll be encouraged to eat lightly during labor. Midwives (who work at birth centers) are generally respectful of a woman's body knowing what it needs. They may suggest you not tackle a cheeseburger or a pan of lasagna, since nausea and slow digestion are very common during labor. Instead, try toast, crackers and cheese, fruit, soup, eggs—y'know, light stuff. If you're not hungry, just keep sipping liquids. If you're queasy, stick to ice chips and wait until you're feeling better.

If you're in the hospital, you're probably not going to be allowed to eat during labor. That's because every labor patient is considered a potential candidate for an epidural and for surgery. Both epidurals and surgical pain relief are provided by anesthetists or anesthesiologists whose main domain is the operating room. Surgery is safer when the patient has an empty stomach, because if she vomits (it happens sometimes during surgery), she risks inhaling chunks into her lungs, which can lead to pneumonia.

Therefore, if you're in labor in the hospital, the anesthetist wants to make sure you're ready to go to the OR at a moment's notice. She doesn't want you vomiting during surgery, so no food for you, hungry mama. You may get to have juice, popsicles, and clear liquids as long as you don't have an epidural. As soon as your epidural goes in, though, it's nothing by mouth except for maybe ice chips or small sips of water.

Is there any way around this hunger strike? Some hospitals are more enlightened than others, and many nurses, midwives, and doctors are pretty lenient. Some are even happy to order you a sandwich, but this isn't the norm. If you're hungry while you're in labor, my best tip (as long as you don't have an epidural—then, seriously, follow the rules) is to pack a lunchbox with easily digestible foods and don't ask for permission. Oh, and eat something before you go to the hospital.

CHAPTER 10

Labor Pains

After all the months of planning and prepping for labor, you still don't
really know what the big event is going to be like unless you have been
there before. And even if you have had a baby before, every labor is
different. This chapter tells it like it is—the the glory and guts of labor,
plus information about your pain management options and the realities
of labor.

The biggest difference between your first and second labors (or third, or fourth . . .)

Every labor consists of the same predictable stages and processes: contractions, dilation, pushing, and eventually, birth. But as similar as they
all are, every labor is different, and individual women have very individual experiences. Even in the same mother, no two labors are alike. The
biggest difference between first and subsequent labors is that first-time
mothers' bodies are untested. Second-time (third, fourth . . . whatever)
mom-bodies know what they're doing.

In general, the first labor tends to be the longest and toughest for
most women. The uterus has to figure out how to do the big job of evict-
ing the baby it has held onto so tightly for nine months. As the baby
descends into the birth canal, the cervix has to learn to dilate and the
pelvic bones and muscles have to stretch and soften and allow baby to
pass through. Then, as the baby emerges, the vagina and perineum have
to stretch and release. It isn't easy, and the learning curve is huge.

The second labor tends to be shorter for most women, though not necessarily less intense. The uterus has muscle memory and remembers what to do. Mothers remember what the experience is like, too, and are less shocked by what their body goes through. They may not be in any less pain, but they know they endured it the first time, they know what pain management measures work for them, and they tend to be more confident that they'll be OK.

With the third labor, it's anyone's guess as to whether it will be shorter, longer, or similar to the second birth. The uterus may be less toned than it was with babies one and two, since it has been stretched out a couple of times. Or it may be a powerfully trained muscle that's ready to flex its stuff. You never know with the third.

Fourth, fifth, sixth . . . these mothers tend to pop their babies out fairly "easily." Labor still hurts like hell, but the process tends to be faster, and pushing is usually easier. The uterus of a "grand multip" (that's medical speak for a mother who's had a bunch of babies) is sometimes big and boggy (flabby, soft, not firm), and if it can't clamp down well after birth and delivery of the placenta, the mother may experience heavy blood loss (hemorrhage). In hospital births, a post-placenta dose of oxytocin or Methergine is usually enough to prevent serious complications.

I say "in general" and "tend to" because labor doesn't always fall into a predictable pattern. Some first-time mothers speed through labor and some second-time mothers dawdle. The timing, pace, and process are a complicated dance between mom's body, baby's body, and the conditions under which labor is taking place. If mom is mobile during labor instead of stuck in bed, her labor may progress more smoothly and quickly. If she's getting contraction-inducing medications, it may go faster than if she's laboring under the power of her own hormones. If she's dehydrated, her uterus may contract less efficiently. If her baby is very large, her uterus may have to work harder and longer.

A pregnant nurse I worked with in the maternity unit came into the hospital in labor with her first baby. Her first contraction started at midnight and her baby was born before 2 A.M. Her second baby came in less than an hour, and the only reason he wasn't born on her living room rug was because labor started while she was at work, taking care of another woman in labor. You can bet her patient was impressed by her birthing prowess and a little bit jealous that she got the whole thing over with in record time. When this nurse had baby number three, though, labor seemed to drag on forever—at least from her perspective. It took four whole hours for her to deliver her baby. Like I said, there's just no telling.

How bad is labor, anyway?

I know there are women who consider labor a pleasurable, powerful experience. Some even describe it as "orgasmic." Some women say contractions aren't painful at all, but merely intense. I've actually witnessed labors like these a time or two. I've also been at the bedside for thousands and thousands of other labors—ones not described as pleasurable, merely intense, or the least bit orgasmic. They're described with less favorable words, ranging from "bad" to "an f'ing nightmare." I'm sorry. I wish I could say it ain't so, but for the vast majority of women, labor is pretty darn painful. More painful than anything else.

Using a pain scale from 1 to 10—1 being virtually no pain and 10 being the worst pain imaginable—most women describe contractions during active labor as being an 11. The pain doesn't just live in the uterus, but often extends to the hips, back, thighs, perineum, and intestines, and it is often accompanied by nausea and vomiting. It's a total body experience.

When labor is really active, there's a minute or so of pain followed by a minute of rest, and this cycle goes on for hours, sometimes even days. It's messy, sweaty, bloody business, and I wouldn't be doing you any favors if I were to sugarcoat it and say it's not that hard. It's hard for women in the United States, hard for women in Africa, hard for women in Peru, hard for women all over the world.

There—we've gotten the god-awful truth out of the way. Now, let's talk about how to dial down the bad. Most of the bad revolves around pain. Here in the United States, women have three basic ways of managing pain (more details on pages 131 to 136):

1: Go natural, which means no narcotics or epidural. Hot baths, showers, and compresses, deep relaxation techniques, and massage help a lot.

2: Get some pain medication through an IV. This is a popular choice during labor for women who need some relief but don't want to have an epidural. Most women say these drugs take the edge off and make pain more bearable, but the effect doesn't generally last for more than an hour or two.

3: Get an epidural. About 65 percent[1] of American women receive epidurals during labor, which consists of an injection of numbing medication into the space surrounding the spinal column. It takes the pain away completely in most cases, but also leaves women unable to walk or move around on their own until the epidural is discontinued and has worn off. It's the most popular method of labor pain relief in America. Epidural rates are higher at some hospitals than others, based on varying patient populations, availability of anesthetists, and patient-physician preferences. (Learn more about epidurals on page 136.)

In the United Kingdom, only about 30 percent of women use epidurals.[2] In Canada the rate is about 50 percent. What do these countries have that American women don't? Nitrous oxide (aka gas and air or laughing gas), which dials contraction pain down considerably without the shot in the back or complete numbness. They also have midwifery-based care and greater access to birthing tubs, both of which are associated with less use of pain medications.

Nitrous oxide was popular in the United States prior to the 1960s, when epidurals became available. This odorless, colorless, patient-administered gas was safe, widely used, and effective through all stages of labor. When epidurals came on the scene, though, and profits from epidural use went up, gas went out the window. Now very few hospitals make nitrous oxide available, but since about 2007, it has been making a comeback. Why? Because it provides an excellent way to dial down the bad and gives women a middle path between an all-natural birth and an epidural. If you live in a major city, ask your midwife or doctor if your hospital has nitrous oxide. It's not available everywhere yet, but its use at major hospitals is increasing.

What else can you do to dial down the bad? Dial up the good. There are many aspects of labor that are, believe it or not, wonderful. Women who experience labor as a positive and beautiful event often describe it as a spiritual and physical experience, almost like an elite athletic event. They celebrate what their body can do. They honor the sacredness of welcoming their baby. They enjoy the intimacy of the experience with their partner. They create as mellow a vibe as possible and immerse themselves in the experience, knowing it's something they'll do only a few times in their life. They use meditation and relaxation techniques and ask for soothing touch and massage. They make the best of an extremely challenging situation, and then something amazing happens— it's not that bad, and in fact, it's kinda good.

Pain management 101— everything from deep breaths to epidurals, and how to take it one step at a time

Now that we've seen how widely the pain management pendulum can swing, let's break down the methods, from most natural to most medical.

Breathing

Gone are the days of the heavily choreographed "hee-hee-hoo-hoo" breathing from Lamaze's early roots. Now any type of patterned, slow, deep breathing will do. The idea is to focus on the breath throughout a contraction to facilitate relaxation. It acts as a type of meditation that focuses the mind on something other than pain, calms the entire body, and, as an extra bonus, increases oxygen flow to boost energy. Does it help? Yes, but it helps more if you practice getting into the deep breathing zone throughout pregnancy. Lamaze, HypnoBirthing, Birthing from

Within, and many hospital-based prenatal education programs will teach you how to breathe like a champ.

Bathtubs

Soaking in hot water (not scalding, but hot is OK) is the best natural pain management technique out there. Fill it as high as it will go, get in, and relax. If you have a Jacuzzi or extra deep tub and can get the water to cover your belly—excellent. If not, bring a bath towel into the tub with you. Get it wet and lay it over your chest, breasts, and belly. Add your favorite breathing technique, and don't be surprised if you dilate more rapidly. Does it help? Yes, absolutely. It may be all you need to get through labor. Many hospital labor units have birthing tubs and Jacuzzis available for laboring patients. Some even have inflatable pools that enable waterbirth.

Hot and cold compresses

When a soak in the tub isn't doable, use washcloths soaked in super-warm water as a compress to ease back pain or a bath towel soaked in hot water draped over the belly for contraction pain. Keep a large bowl and kettle of hot water next to the bed to reheat compresses.

Use washcloths soaked in cold water to cool a hot forehead. When your cold compress gets warm, just twirl it in the air like a lasso to rechill without returning to the sink.

If you're not into getting wet, use an electric heating pad (if your hospital will OK that—some won't) or heat a rice sock in the microwave (fill a tube sock with dry rice and stitch up the opening, or buy a rice sock premade) and apply it to sore muscles.

Birthing balls and stools

While they aren't technically used to ease pain, they do help laboring women get into positions that facilitate labor, keep them out of bed, and take some pressure off the back. Do they help with pain? Yes, and even more, they're an all-around excellent, functional labor tool that supports natural birth.

Relaxation techniques

Are the tips you'll learn in your hospital-based prenatal education enough? Probably not. If you really want a natural birth, you're going to need to go deeper. Whether it's Lamaze, Leboyer, Bradley, Grantly Dick-Read, HypnoBirthing, or another of the countless other relaxation and natural birth philosophies out there, the key to having a natural birth is being able to relax deeply during contractions. We're not talking about simply chilling out. We're talking about a level and depth of relaxation that takes skill, focus, and training. Deep breathing, deep relaxation, and deep meditation often work in tandem, and different techniques and schools of natural birth philosophy use different approaches to achieve relaxation. I recommend that you check out a couple of philosophies/techniques until you find one that seems feasible and doable. Then start practicing as far in advance of your due date as possible. Do these methods work? For many women, absolutely. I'm a big fan of HypnoBirthing because it seems to work the best, though that may be just because it's popular in the hospitals I've worked in. Other techniques may work better in other hospitals. Go with whatever philosophy clicks with you.

Meditation

Like breathing and conscious relaxation techniques, the various forms of meditation work on the same level to achieve deep relaxation, focus, and detachment from pain. Visualization is another form of meditation that many people find helpful. Pick a vision or an image that's relaxing—aka "your happy place"—and maintain total focus on it throughout contractions. Meditation is an excellent labor tool, but not one you can pull out of your pocket without having practiced for a while in advance. Most people find it challenging enough to still the mind without the distraction of hard contractions. Find a meditation teacher in the Buddhist or Tibetan community or through a meditation center and take a few lessons. Then practice daily. As a bonus, if you continue your meditation practice after birth, it'll help improve many areas of your health and life, not the least of which is parenting. Does it help? Oh yes, it does—it helps everything. Go for the Zen, baby.

Hypnosis

Like meditation, breathing, and relaxation, hypnosis can direct your mind away from pain. You'll need to be able to use self-hypnosis techniques, rather than relying on a hypnotist to drop you into this deep relaxation state. As already mentioned, HypnoBirthing is great. Does it work? Sure it does, but you have to learn the techniques and practice, practice, practice.

Massage

Your husband, partner, doula, or nurse (if she has time) can massage sore muscles in your back, neck, arms, and legs. Don't massage the belly—most women find that really annoying. If you're having back labor (serious pain in the low back), massage or applied pressure to the painful area is a godsend. The reason massage eases pain is the same as all the other techniques mentioned so far—it helps you relax. But a lot of women find that being touched, rubbed, or massaged during labor is overwhelming. They're already feeling as much sensation as they can stand, thankyouverymuch, and the extra input of massage is irritating. Tell your masseuse in advance that when you say, "Knock that off," it's nothing personal.

Movement and positioning

Sometimes the best way to ease pain and reset your ability to tolerate labor is to change position. If you've been sitting a while, move to the bed and lie on your side. If you've been lying down a while, switch to all fours. Go for a walk, practice some yoga (no inversions—duh), rock in the rocker, use the birthing ball—just move it. The more you move, the better able your body will be to facilitate labor. This only works, though, if you don't have an epidural, which numbs you from the waist down and impedes standing, walking, and other movement.

IV narcotics

Opiate medications like Stadol, fentanyl, morphine, Nubain, and Demerol are the drugs of choice often used to take the edge off during labor. They provide relaxation, relief from anxiety, and some degree of pain relief. Some women get a lot of relief from a shot of one of these drugs in their IV—as much as a couple of hours or more of almost total pain relief. More often, women get "some" relief for an hour or so. Although the pain doesn't really go away, IV drugs take the edge off or, as many women describe it, "make it so you just don't care that much anymore." The first dose works the best. All subsequent doses will probably be less effective, since pain amplifies as labor progresses and the body's narcotic receptors fill up. If your care providers think your baby will be born in less than an hour after you would receive a dose, they probably won't give you one. Babies can suffer respiratory depression because narcotics cross the placenta and transfer to them. If your baby is born shortly after a narcotic is administered to you and if he's having trouble breathing, he may receive a shot of Narcan to counteract the effects. If you need more than two doses of IV narcotic during labor, chances are you need an epidural. Your nurse may or may not offer you a repeat dose of narcotics. If you feel like your dose has worn off and you want another one, don't hesitate to ask for more. If it's too soon for a repeat dose or your nurse thinks your baby is coming too quickly, she'll let you know.

Nitrous oxide

This odorless, colorless gas is inhaled by mom through a mask. It's also called "gas and air," or laughing gas. Nitrous oxide knocks the edge off contraction pain during all stages of labor. It does not transfer through the placenta and is entirely controlled by the patient. Women who use it say it works really well and in many cases is all they need during labor. It's used in dentist offices and maternity wards all over the world and was popular here in the United States prior to the 1960s. It's not currently available in most American hospitals, but it's beginning to make a comeback as American hospitals begin looking abroad to countries with better maternal health stats than the United States has. Most of these countries also have much lower epidural rates than the United States has, and many women find that by using nitrous oxide they get enough relief to be able to avoid needing an epidural. It's been considered a safe drug for laboring mothers since the 1950s and is used in a majority of birth facilities in Europe, Australia, Canada, and the UK.

Epidurals

These are widely available at all hospitals that provide maternity services. They're administered by a certified registered nurse anesthetist or an anesthesiologist. See the next section, "Epidural 101," for complete details.

After delivery, you can use oral pain medications like ibuprofen (Advil), acetaminophen (Tylenol), Percocet, and Vicodin, but none of them are effective or appropriate for tackling labor pain.

Will you need all of these pain management options while you're in labor? Probably not, but you should have a handful of natural techniques at the ready, as well as a solid working knowledge of how narcotics and epidurals work, too. As I mentioned earlier, you really don't know what labor's going to be like until you're smack dab in the middle of it.

Epidural 101—how it works, who puts it in, why it takes a while, and why you can't custom-order it

Epidurals are crazy popular in America, primarily because we don't have many other effective options for pain relief during labor besides natural techniques (which are effective for some, not effective for others) and narcotics (which don't work well enough or long enough for many women). On average, between 65 and 70 percent of American mothers use epidurals to give birth, and in some hospitals epidural rates are as high as 95 percent. That's because they work really well at eliminating most, if not all, labor and birth pain.

Epidurals are categorized as regional anesthesia because they block pain in a specific region of the body. They're used for many kinds of surgeries, including C-sections, as well as for labor pain relief. Unlike general anesthesia, which knocks women out, epidurals eliminate pain but allow the patient to be awake, alert, and comfortable.

Epidurals are administered by certified registered nurse anesthetists (CRNA—registered nurses with advanced training and a master's degree in administering anesthesia) or anesthesiologists (medical doctors who specialize in anesthesia). The procedure involves threading a tube in between the vertebrae and infusing numbing medication into the area that surrounds the spinal cord. It works by blocking nerve impulses that transmit pain sensations in areas of the body below the epidural insertion site. Since epidurals are inserted into the mid-to-lower section of the spine, all sensations below that point are blocked—not only to the uterus but also to the legs and feet.

Once the epidural tubing is inserted, the patient can receive a continuous dose of numbing medication, which should leave her comfortable throughout the duration of her labor and birth or surgery. Once the medication is turned off or discontinued, the numbing effect gradually goes away, and most women can feel their lower body parts again within a couple of hours.

Getting an epidural isn't fast, like popping a pill or getting a shot. It takes a while to prepare and administer an epidural, and certain procedures have to be followed to the letter (no shortcuts) in order to be safe and effective. There has to be a doctor or midwife's order for the patient to receive an epidural. Consents have to be signed, lab tests ordered, blood drawn, an IV started, and at least a full liter of fluid has to be infused. Then the anesthetist has to be called in (hopefully he's already in the hospital and not at home), and the patient has to receive a pre-epidural consultation that includes an explanation of the procedure, potential complications and side effects, and a health Q&A. Once all that has taken place, the patient will go to the bathroom to empty her bladder and then get ready to receive her epidural.

The procedure itself is usually called "uncomfortable," but it's not as bad as many patients think it will be. It's done under sterile technique, to minimize chances of infection in the area where the epidural is administered. Once the anesthetist has set up all his equipment and donned sterile gloves, the nurse will help the patient get into either a side-lying position or take a seat on the edge of her bed (positioning is per anesthetist's choice, not the patient's, and is based on her training and technique and the patient's anatomy). The patient will be asked to curl up (like a shrimp) with her back humped out (like a mad cat) and to remain still throughout the procedure.

Being able to stay still is a real sticking point (pun totally intended). When patients can't or won't remain still, the anesthetist can't do her job safely. She's sticking a needle into your spine, after all, and it's a very exacting technique. You don't want her messing that up. When the patient is so uncomfortable she's unable to stay in position, she may be offered a dose of narcotic pain medication in her IV to help her relax. Once in a while, a patient is just plain jumpy or squirmy or doesn't get it that still means STILL! Most anesthetists are extremely patient and willing to help patients understand what they need to do. The nurse is there to help the patient stay in position. But every now and then there's a patient who won't settle down, and the only thing the anesthetist can do is decline to do the procedure. It's not safe to poke a long needle into a moving target.

Next, the anesthetist will cleanse the patient's back with a cleaning solution (usually Betadine, which looks like brown soap and may temporarily leave an orange residue on the skin) and then put a sterile drape (tape-lined sterile paper) on the patient's back. The next step is the painful part. The anesthetist will inject numbing medication (probably Lidocaine) into the skin and tissues right around the insertion site. This stings like crazy for about 10 seconds. She'll probably do more than one injection, but it's usually only the first one that hurts. Patients say it feels like a bee sting, but the sensation goes away quickly. After that, most patients think getting an epidural feels weird, but not actually painful.

Once the skin is numb, the CRNA will use a very long needle (you may not want to look at it in advance, and you may want to give your partner a heads-up—it's a big one) that's threaded with an epidural catheter (a very thin plastic tube). She'll insert it between two spinal vertebrae and advance it slowly until she feels a loss of resistance indicating she's found the right spot. She can't see where she's going once she's through the skin, and she wants to be absolutely certain about where the needle and catheter go—therefore the need for absolute stillness.

Once she thinks she has the needle in the right location, she'll inject a small amount of air through a syringe into the needle to make sure. She wants the needle to go to a fluid-filled area (the epidural space) outside the spinal cord. If she's sure the needle is where she wants it to be, she'll then pull back on the syringe to see if any blood or spinal fluid returns into the syringe. If it does, she relocates the needle. If it doesn't (which is what she wants), then she'll inject a test dose of medication while the nurse checks the patient's pulse rate. If the patient's pulse speeds up, that indicates the needle is in a blood vessel and needs to be repositioned. If the pulse remains steady, however, then the CRNA removes the needle but leaves the catheter in place. Then she'll inject a dose of medication that will begin to make the patient go numb. It will take as long as 20 minutes before the patient is truly out of pain, but once she's received that initial dose, each contraction after that should be gradually less and less painful. After a few minutes, the nurse may ask, "How did that contraction feel?" and the patient will probably answer, "What contraction?" It's that good.

After that first dose of medication is delivered, the nurse will check the patient's blood pressure every few minutes until she's sure it's stable and then every 15 minutes. An epidural can make mom's blood pressure drop suddenly, which is why we preload patients with a liter or more of IV fluid. We know this can happen, and we know how to fix it, but we also know that low blood pressure in mom can affect the baby, so we're vigilant to make sure both mother and baby are fine. That's why you'll get lots of blood pressure checks.

The CRNA will tape the heck out of the catheter, which remains in the back for as long as the patient needs the epidural. It's a lot of tape— seriously. We want to make sure that little tube stays put. This brings up the other uncomfortable part of having an epidural—having the tape removed after you've delivered your baby and no longer need your epidural. Think of it like ripping off a massive adhesive bandage or like getting your back waxed.

The catheter is hooked up to IV tubing that's attached to an IV bag of medication that keeps you numb as long as needed. It's infused in a small, continuous dose and regulated by the CRNA through an electronic pump. Usually that continuous dose keeps you comfortable, but if you feel breakthrough pain, the CRNA can come back in and give you a bolus (extra dose) that should make you comfy again quickly.

Occasionally, an epidural doesn't work as planned. Remember, the anesthetist can't see where the catheter goes once it's past the skin. If it runs along one side of the nerve bundle that supplies the uterus, you may get one-sided relief, or a "window" of pain while the rest of your abdomen is numb. In that case, the CRNA may fiddle with the catheter or completely redo the epidural procedure to get better pain relief. This does not mean your anesthetist is lame. It's just the way it goes with these things. Every woman's anatomy is a little different, and every anesthetist has her own technique. If she's tried a couple of times and just can't get it right, then ask for another anesthetist to give it a try. It's possible that your anatomy and your anesthetist's technique aren't a good match. If your anesthetist is the only one available, you'll have to choose whether to have her keep trying or forgo an epidural.

There are a few different types of epidurals that all work more or less the same.

The standard epidural uses a combination of drugs (a narcotic mixed with an anesthetic/numbing medication) injected through a pump or by hand. This makes the abdomen, back, pelvis, vagina, and legs feel heavy and numb. Often the first dose of medication is stronger than the rest (to get mom out of pain ASAP), and when that wears off after an hour or so, feeling may or may not return to the legs for a while. That doesn't mean pain will come back. The continuous infusion will take care of that. The goal of an epidural is to dial down the patient's pain level on a 1-to-10 scale to about a 2 or 3. Most of the time, it takes it to a 0 or 1.

A combined spinal-epidural (SCE) works the same, but the first dose of medication is fast-acting and injected into the intrathecal space (the outermost membrane covering the spinal cord) and the epidural space. Sometimes this first dose lasts long enough that mom won't need any other medication. It works faster than a standard epidural. If mom needs more medication for a longer period of time, she'll be hooked up to a continuous drip. Most moms have a bit more mobility with a CSE and less leg numbness.

A light epidural takes the edge off the pain but the patient can still feel pressure and move her legs. She may also still feel some level of pain with contractions, but nowhere near what she'd feel without an epidural. This is sometimes called a "walking epidural," but that's an overstatement. It's not likely mom will have enough feeling and mobility in her legs to be able to walk the halls even with a light epidural.

As mentioned earlier, you'll get the type of epidural your anesthetist can administer to your body safely and effectively and the one that's most appropriate for your labor. Don't expect that you can order one up in precisely the style you want. It doesn't work that way. This is a go-with-the-flow situation.

From the moment a mom says she wants one to the moment she no longer feels pain may be as little as a half hour (*if* her paperwork, IV, and lab work are already done and she's already had a preprocedure consultation and an anesthetist is on site and speedy), but more commonly it takes about an hour. Sometimes patients have to wait their turn, especially if the maternity ward is busy and multiple patients need CRNA services. It's not necessarily a situation where patients take a number and get served in order, either. If one mother is moving quickly through labor and in big-time pain and another mother is moving slowly, then the mom with greater need may be served first. If another mom needs emergency surgery and there's only one anesthetist to go around, the rest must wait their turn. That's why I mentioned earlier that every mom should know all her pain management options and a few good natural pain management techniques.

Epidural FAQs

Now that we've covered how epidurals work, how they're inserted, and what you have to do to get one, let's tackle some of the most commonly asked questions about them.

Are epidurals safe?

Epidurals are widely considered safe for moms and babies, but that doesn't mean they aren't without side effects and potential complications. In almost all cases, an epidural is inserted without any hitches. It works like a dream with no residual side effects, and the patient loves it. Once in a while, as mentioned in Epidural 101, a patient may have to go through a couple of attempts before her anesthetist gets it placed in the right location. While any type of invasive procedure has a risk of complications like infection, the risk goes up a teensy bit if the procedure has to be done more than once.

Most women who ask if it's safe have heard stories about someone who had an epidural and was left with permanent back pain. Or maybe they heard it causes paralysis. While backache (for a short period of time) may result, paralysis doesn't. Usually when I hear about the epidural-paralysis connection, it's said to have taken place in another country. I can't speak to the veracity of that situation except to say, if the person administering an epidural doesn't know what the heck he or she is doing, then paralysis is a possibility. Here in the United States (and in almost all places where epidurals are routinely administered), anesthetists are trained, certified, licensed, vetted, and highly skilled. Don't worry about it. It's pretty darn safe.

What kind of side effects do epidurals have?

Here's the rundown of things we see fairly often.

Hypotension (low blood pressure)
Sometimes epidural medication causes mom's blood pressure to bottom out. It has to do with the way nerves and blood vessels respond to the medication. This can make mom feel lousy (dizzy, nauseated, weak)

and can make baby's heart rate drop. Again, this is why we load mom up with lots of IV fluid in advance of getting an epidural. The cure for hypotension is to give mom more IV fluids, change her position to one that improves circulation, and give her oxygen until her blood pressure improves. Sometimes the anesthetist has to give mom a dose of ephedrine to bump her blood pressure up quickly. Once mom has enough fluid on board, her blood pressure will stabilize.

Nausea and vomiting

This is usually a reaction to low blood pressure. Once mom's blood pressure stabilizes, the nausea should go away. If it doesn't or blood pressure isn't the problem, mom may be treated with antinausea medication. Nausea and vomiting are part of a lot of labors, both with and without epidurals.

Itching

Some of the medication given in an epidural can make moms itchy. About 30 to 50 percent of moms complain of an itchy face, neck, arms, or chest, most often in the first hour or so. If it's really a bother, she can get some anti-itch medication in her IV.

The shivers

Many women experience uncontrollable shivers after their epidural sets up, and no one's exactly sure why. I've heard many explanations for why that happens, including:

- The nerves are misfiring an "I'm super cold" message to the brain.
- It's a reaction to all the IV fluids we dump in before and during the epidural.
- It's hormones (we can blame almost everything on that, right?).
- It's because the body is responding to contractions.
- It's the epidural medications.

Nobody is 100-percent sure it isn't all of the above. But shivering is not dangerous. It's very common, and a heap of heated blankets helps a lot. It usually goes away within an hour.

Ringing in the ears

This also happens when blood pressure drops. If you've ever fainted, you probably experienced this. It goes away when the blood pressure increases.

Fever

Usually a fever is a sign of infection, but with epidurals that's not always the case. Approximately 20 percent of women get a fever with their epidural, but it's often hard to pinpoint whether that's because of the epidural, dehydration, or an infection brewing (especially if her water has broken). She may be treated with Tylenol and an antibiotic.

Headache

I've mentioned before that epidurals are what we call "blind procedures." The anesthetist can't see where the needle and catheter are going once they're past the skin. If he pierces the spinal cord, spinal fluid can leak out. This can cause a horrible headache that can last several days or longer after delivery. It happens to only about 1 percent of women, but that 1 percent are miserable. A "spinal headache" can be treated with a procedure called a "blood patch," where blood is drawn from the patient (just like with a lab test) and injected into the spine where the epidural was placed. It forms a clot that seals the leak and stops the cause of pain. The pain itself can be treated with pain medication like morphine, Vicodin, or Percocet.

Difficulty urinating

Quite a few women who have an epidural need a urinary catheter inserted while they're in labor (or after). Since they can't get up to go to the bathroom with numb legs and they often can't release their urinary sphincter (it's anesthetized, too) to pee in a bedpan, we empty their bladder for them. We'll do that by inserting a onetime catheter through the urethra and into the bladder (don't worry, you won't feel it), and once the bladder is emptied, remove the catheter right away. Or we place a Foley catheter, which stays in the bladder for as long as we need it. Catheters can (not commonly) cause a urinary tract infection, and they can "confuse" the sphincter. After the epidural is removed, the numbing effect has worn off, and the patient is able to get up to go to the bathroom, she may still feel like she can't pee. It's temporary, and while occasionally it requires putting in another catheter, more often nurses use "make you pee" tricks that work like a charm. Just like at middle-school slumber parties, putting your hand in warm water often does the trick. So does listening to running water, having running water poured over your perineum, or sniffing peppermint oil. Weird, right?

There's a mixed bag of other side effects associated with epidurals that we see occasionally. They include infection, bleeding, long-term backache and headache, difficulty walking for more than a day after the epidural is discontinued, and, very, very rarely, seizures and death. These two happen only if epidural medication is injected directly into the bloodstream. I have never seen this happen, and I've taken care of thousands and thousands of patients with epidurals.

Do epidurals slow down labor?

Yes, they can slow down labor, but usually only for a little while. Whenever labor hormones (oxytocin) are diluted (with lots of pre-epidural IV fluids), contractions can slow down or become less strong. That's why it's not uncommon for contractions to disappear for a while immediately after an epidural is started. They'll be back, but you may have a longer labor than you would have without one. An epidural also decreases your mobility. Women who walk, squat, rock, sit, lean, and move around during labor usually have a shorter labor than women with an epidural who are stuck in bed.

A slow or stopped labor also happens sometimes when an epidural is put in before labor is really active. Sometimes women get an epidural too early, when they aren't actually in real labor. They may be in early labor or prodromal labor and it may hurt, but their uterus, brain, and all the rest of it aren't fully committed to doing the job at hand. When labor stops altogether, sometimes it has to be charged back up with Pitocin and/or rupture of membranes. Getting an epidural before you're in active labor isn't ideal, but some women are in such great pain in early labor that they need an epidural early. Many doctors and mid-wives allow their patients to get an epidural at any point during labor because they know they can always give labor a jump with Pitocin.

Can epidurals speed labor up?

Absolutely! I've seen it happen hundreds of times when a woman gets stuck at a certain dilation for hours. She's painful and miserable and can't catch a break between contractions. When she finally gets an epidural and the pain is gone, she usually goes to sleep (because she's exhausted, not because the epidural knocks her out—it doesn't) and becomes relaxed. Once mom is able to rest and relax, her muscles relax, too (though her uterus keeps contracting), and her cervix is able to dilate. Pretty soon she's fully dilated and ready to push. That's what happened to me with my first baby. I was determined to go natural, but after 25 hours of active labor I got stuck at 4 centimeters for what seemed like days. I finally surrendered to an epidural. I took a two-hour nap and woke up 10 centimeters dilated. My baby was born an hour later. Sometimes, an epidural is a freakin' miracle worker.

Do epidurals increase C-section rates?

Studies indicate that epidurals can contribute to increased C-section rates and to increased need for forceps and vacuum extractors, probably because an epidural can reduce a woman's ability to push effectively.

Stories from lots of women and midwives also indicate that when women spend their labor lying down or in one position, it impacts the normal physiologic process of labor, which may lead to a C-section. I've also seen C-sections happen in response to the fairly common blood pressure drop that can cause baby's heart rate to plummet. While most of the time that's easily fixed with more IV fluid and a little ephedrine for mom, if baby's heart rate doesn't respond quickly, nobody will hesitate to run to the OR.

Is it better to go natural than to have an epidural?

Better for some, not better for others. It really depends on how labor is going, how the epidural affects you, and if, in the end, you were satisfied with how it all played out. There are some definite advantages to going natural in terms of being able to work with your body's natural physiology, stay mobile, and push well. There are some definite advantages to having an epidural, too—namely, you don't feel horrible pain. For somewhere around 65 percent of American women, that's a great big thumbs-up.

Am I a wimp if I wanted to go natural but caved in and got an epidural?

Oh, *hell* no. You're right on par with a grand majority of women. Labor hurts—a lot. If you're not into the word "hurts" (some birth philosophies aren't), then we'll say it like this: Labor is really intense. Super intense. If it's way more intense than you can stand, nobody's judging you. Do what you have to do to get through labor. For some women, the difference between sticking to their natural goals and getting an epidural is the difference between having a horrible, violent, traumatic birth and one that's rather peaceful and lovely. Now, most natural births *aren't* horrible, violent, and traumatic. Most of them, when mom can handle the "intensity," *are* peaceful and lovely—but not all of them. Some are downright horrid, and getting an epidural is a great and wonderful thing. Are you a wimp? No, honey, you're a woman. Use the tools *you* need to get the job done.

Is it ever too late to get an epidural?

In "Epidural 101" I mentioned that it usually takes about an hour (more or less) to have an epidural catheter inserted and another 20 minutes or so for the medication to take effect and reduce pain. If your baby is on her way out, there may not be time to get an epidural. That said, I've helped countless women get an epidural when they were 9 centimeters dilated. It really all depends on the speed of your labor, the availability of an anesthetist, and the time it takes to put the epidural in. If you don't have time, consider yourself lucky that labor is moving that quickly.

What's Pitocin really like?

Here are the questions I'm asked most often about Pitocin:

- Why do I actually need it?

- Is Pitocin as bad as they say? Does it really hurt like labor
  times ten?

Pitocin is a synthetic form of oxytocin, the natural hormone humans
secrete that causes contractions. It also causes milk to flow—and feelings of love to well up. It's often called the feel-good hormone because
it's released when we snuggle and have sex. We secrete it big-time during labor, but nobody calls it the feel-good hormone then.

Why would you need Pitocin?

Most women produce enough oxytocin during labor to have plenty of
contractions that are strong enough to get them all the way through
labor, birth, and then some. Some women, however—those who need
to have their labor induced (started medically) or augmented (powered
up/helped along)—receive Pitocin intravenously to create contractions
for them. Who are these women?

- Women with medical conditions that are best treated by delivering the baby prior to labor starting spontaneously. These conditions include dangerously high blood pressure, preeclampsia, and
  other maternal or fetal illnesses.

- Women with social circumstances that motivate them to request
  induction. This happens a lot, and it shouldn't. There are very few
  social circumstances that warrant the risks of induction.

- Women whose contractions aren't strong enough or frequent
  enough for labor to progress. This doesn't happen often. Most
  women who are in active labor contract plenty, thankyouverymuch. If the doctor or midwife decides labor isn't moving fast
  enough, or mom's not dilating as quickly as the provider wants,
  she may order Pitocin to speed things up. One might argue,
  "Not fast enough for whom?" but few women make that argu-
  ment when their doctor orders the pit.

The biggest difference between a labor that's powered by Pitocin and one that's powered by mom's own hormones (oxytocin) is that with pit, mom's body doesn't have access to the control panel. Pitocin is pumped into the vein through an IV that's attached to a nurse-regulated electronic pump, so it's the nurse (who follows orders and a protocol that spells out how much Pitocin to give) who's in control of when the patient has contractions. Mom's chemical receptors pick up the Pitocin and send it along its way to neurons that tell the uterus to contract. The nurse regulates the dose given through the IV pump to generate contractions approximately every 3 minutes (counting from the beginning of one contraction to the beginning of the next). If Mom has too many contractions, the nurse dials down the infusion. Not enough, she dials it up.

Many women say that having Pitocin makes their contractions a lot stronger and more painful. During inductions, contractions come on more abruptly than they generally do with natural labors. Instead of having mild contractions spaced well apart at the beginning of labor and then becoming closer and stronger over time, inductions can go from zero to sixty in nothing flat. It's not always like that, but it often is.

Pitocin also adds some bite and muscle to contractions. It makes the uterus contract harder to push the baby lower into the birth canal and make the cervix dilate. That's what it's designed to do, but it hurts. Of course, normal labor hurts plenty, too.

Not all women experience Pitocin as worse than normal labor. Many do—that's where the "labor times ten" reputation comes from. My own direct experience is limited to two induced labors (I had normal labors with my first and second babies and Pitocin with my third and fourth). I didn't find labor with Pitocin very different from labor without it. Baby number one was by far my toughest labor—without Pitocin—though admittedly first labors are the most difficult for many women. Baby number two came super fast, but my labor was so powerful and intense it about blew me away (again, no Pitocin). Baby number three was my biggest baby, and he was induced. I'll tell that induction story later, but for the purpose of this discussion, I don't remember his labor being particularly hard. Same with number four, also an induction.

Is Pitocin as bad as they say?

Again, many women say Pitocin is "bad" because it makes their contractions more painful. But ultimately Pitocin is just a tool, and a hard-working one. If you need it in order to get through labor, it's not bad at all.

CHAPTER 11

Other Labor and Delivery Issues

Even smooth labors can include a few bumps. Some are to big deal and others are potentially huge deals. Chances are, the potentially huge deals won't happen to women who have had normal pregnancies, but it's always important to have a full understanding of these issues and to know what to look out for.

Meconium—what does it mean when sh** happens?

Sometimes meconium (aka baby's first poop) is a sign that baby is stressed out and that stress caused him to lose it. Sometimes meconium happens when babies are overdue (they just couldn't hold it any longer). In most cases nobody knows why baby pooped in the uterus and it's absolutely no big deal. If it's super thick and your baby is indicating signs of fetal distress via fetal monitoring (an abnormal heartbeat—too fast, too slow, or an ominous deceleration), that might be a labor game-changer. Your doctor might want to intervene to dilute the meconium (warm IV solution is infused through a catheter into the uterus to give baby a bath and clean out some of the meconium), speed up labor, or opt for a C-section to get your possibly stressed-out baby outta there. Usually, however, it's not thick, but diluted in the amniotic fluid and therefore no big deal.

If you have meconium in your amniotic fluid, there will probably be an extra person or two attending your birth. A respiratory tech, an anesthetist, or a pediatrician may come to your delivery to make sure your baby doesn't inhale meconium into her lungs. When your baby's head is delivered, your provider may tell you to stop pushing so he can suction out her nose and mouth before her body is delivered and before she takes her first breath. When baby is delivered, she may be handed off to the pediatrician, nurse, respiratory tech, or anesthetist as gently as possible to prevent stimulation that will cause her to gasp. Then a more thorough suctioning may be done to make sure there's no meconium in her airway. If they can see down the throat and determine there's nothing there, then the drama's over. Baby will then be dried and handed over to mom.

Babies often take their first breath before they're suctioned, and usually they're absolutely fine. Meconium happens, and it doesn't have to be a big deal. In some cases (not very many, but it happens), babies inhale meconium into their lungs, which can cause pneumonia. If baby shows any signs of respiratory compromise, a fever, fast heart rate, poor color, or inability to eat, she'll make a trip to the nursery for further evaluation. If an X-ray, blood tests, and a pediatric exam determine she's sick, she'll receive oxygen support and antibiotics in the NICU.

I want to restate, this doesn't happen all that often, even though meconium in amniotic fluid happens kind of a lot. Some women think that if they see meconium, that means they're having a big screaming emergency. They probably aren't. They're most likely just having a normal variation on labor. I strongly advise women not to buy into the idea that variations on a normal theme are a reason to freak out. Normal variations, like a little meconium in your fluid, do not mean your labor is abnormal and therefore needs to be fixed. We've gotten into trouble in recent years thinking that we have to intervene in any circumstance that lands outside of a very narrow definition of what constitutes "normal" labor. Every few years it seems like we shift the margins and decide some formerly normal issue is "abnormal."

After decades of "fixing" every little thing, and discovering we're messing up an awful lot of maternal health care, we're coming to realize that not everything different is abnormal, broken, or an emergency or a crisis. Seriously, the less drama you bring to your labor the better. I think that's what I mean by "meconium happens."

The big push—how to do it if you don't have an urge, and how to avoid pushing too hard

I spent decades in hospital labor and delivery units telling countless women how to push, and I'm here to tell you, I wish I hadn't. I wish it had occurred to me that all those women I told to *hold their breath, push like crazy to a count of ten, grab another breath and push again, another breath . . . another ten,* actually could have done as good a job or better without me bossing them around.

I participated in what's often called *coached pushing* for years. That was our culture, because the goal was to get the baby out ASAP before mom got too tired and doctors got impatient. At some point in recent years, somebody finally thought to ask why we did things that way. OK, that's not quite right—many midwives had been asking what all that bossing around was about for a long time. Why weren't we just telling women to do their thing, whatever that thing was? Why were we prescribing this one-style-fits-all pushing technique instead of letting women's bodies be their guide? Oh, you know why—because we medical folks always think we know better than our patients how to manage their bodies. I want to go on record here, saying, *Sorry about that.* You know when you're ready to push better than I do.

If you don't have an epidural, your body will let you know it's go time by sending you an urge so strong you can't ignore it. I think the whole coached pushing thing must have started when epidurals became popular. If you're numb, it's hard to know when you're ready to push. Or maybe coached pushing was invented to give dads something to do and a way to feel involved. Whatever. Mom's the expert here, and it's time for us to quit being so bossy in the delivery room.

Most women, when allowed to push their own way, start pushing at the peak of a contraction and then bear down with short, frequent bursts. They tend to breathe normally or exhale with pushing. With coached pushing, nurses tell moms to hold their breath and aim for three long pushes to a count of ten starting from as soon as the contraction begins to build.

We've spent decades telling women they have to push as soon as they're 10 centimeters dilated, whether or not they feel an urge. We start counting that as the beginning of second stage, and the clock starts ticking. If after two or three hours (or a whole lot less in many cases) of active pushing mom hasn't delivered, we start intervening with forceps, vacuum extractor, or C-section. But who says we have to start pushing before mom feels like it?

What happens if you don't feel an urge to push? As long as mom and baby are both safe and well, there's really no urgency about when to start pushing. In fact, mom's uterus and baby's body will do most of the work without her pushing. If she does not have an epidural, the urge to push will be overwhelming. She'll feel like she must bear down, and at this point, if she works with her body's cues, she'll probably push very effectively and for a lot less time than if she'd been coached to start pushing earlier.

If she has an epidural, she probably won't feel it when she reaches 10 centimeters. The process of baby moving through the birth canal will happen without her feeling it and without her active participation. At some point, though, she will probably feel pressure in her vagina and an urge to push. If she never feels this urge, then at some point someone will do a vaginal exam. When the baby is so low in the vagina that you don't have to reach very far to feel it (or better yet, you can see the head emerging), then mom can be encouraged to push. This more natural approach is called laboring down, which allows the normal labor process to bring baby down through the vagina.

Which approach works better? It depends on whom you ask and what studies you read. Some studies indicate there are no benefits to coached pushing and no adverse outcomes from letting mom's push on their own.[1] Other studies indicate the longer second stage lasts, the worse outcomes for moms and babies. Still other studies say that coached pushing can result in urinary[2] and pelvic floor problems for moms, more perineal bruising and tearing, increased maternal and fetal fatigue, and higher rates of forceps,[3] vacuum extractor, and C-section deliveries.

Some women do need a little support, feedback, and guidance when they're unable to push effectively, but most women don't fall into that category. Most women, if left to their own instincts, will push their baby out in the way that works best for their bodies. I think there's wisdom in leaving Mother Nature alone to do her business. When we do, babies wiggle down in ways that are gentler and more efficient than anything we medical experts can think up. Let's save coached pushing for those few cases that require it instead of making all labors one-push-fits-all.

Vacuums, forceps, and other tools of the trade

What do you do when baby gets stuck, or when baby is almost there, so close to being born you can easily touch him, but he just can't make the last little stretch of his birth journey? Sometimes the answer is to go in after him and help the little guy out. That may mean your doctor does an assisted vaginal delivery and uses a vacuum extractor or forceps.

Assisted vaginal deliveries account for about 5 percent of all births—4 percent use vacuum extractors and 1 percent use forceps. A midwife can use a vacuum, but only doctors use forceps. It used to be far more common for doctors to use these tools to rescue stuck babies, but nowadays C-sections are increasingly the go-to procedure. In fact, some young obstetricians say their training barely skimmed over forceps and vacuums in favor of surgery. That's because these tools can cause fetal injury if used improperly and because C-sections have become a much more widely accepted way of birth for mothers and providers.

The vacuum extractor uses a suction cup device and a handheld pump to grip baby's head and guide him through the birth canal. It's used only when baby is extremely low in the birth canal already and in a good birth position. The suction cup is made of soft, flexible plastic.

It's applied to the crown of baby's head, and when mom has a contraction, the nurse pumps the vacuum until it achieves a seal. As mom pushes, the provider gently pulls on a handle attached to the suction cup and guides the head out of the vagina. If the seal breaks and the suction cup pops off, it can be reapplied, but only twice. After that, it's considered risky to continue putting pressure on baby's head. Vacuums can cause bruising and occasionally even hematomas on baby's head, but generally, they're quite safe and effective. When bruising does occur, babies tend to recover quickly.

Forceps look like long-handled salad tongs. They come in two pieces and fit together to provide a traction device. The doctor slides each piece (one at a time) into the vagina on either side of baby's head. Once she's sure she has the forceps in the position she wants, as mom pushes the doctor pulls gently on the forceps and baby's head to ease baby out of the vagina. Forceps can cause facial and cranial bruising or abrasions, temporary nerve damage, and in very rare cases (really, really rare) skull damage. Forceps are more painful for the mom and have more potential for causing vaginal tears and lacerations than a vacuum, because they are wedged inside the vagina. For that reason, some doctors prefer their patients get spinal anesthesia or an epidural before they use forceps. (Epidurals and spinals are very similar procedures, but spinals work faster, wear off faster, and don't require a catheter to remain in the back.)

Some of the other effective tools of the trade don't involve instruments at all:

- Positioning: Often all a stuck baby needs is for mom to change position. When mom simply switches from lying on one side to lying on the other or moves to a hands-and-knees or squatting position, it opens up enough space in the pelvis that baby can maneuver better.

- Oil is crazy-effective (kind of like putting lotion on your hand to get a stuck ring off) at helping babies slide right out. The nurse, doctor, or midwife can use mineral oil or olive oil, poured inside the vaginal opening, to lubricate the birth canal and to assist in perineal massage, which can help tissues stretch.

What causes babies to get stuck in the first place? Sometimes babies aren't actually stuck and, if given a bit more time, they'd find their way out unassisted. But sometimes baby's head doesn't line up perfectly with mom's pelvis (think oval peg, round hole). Sometimes mom can't push effectively because she has an epidural or she's exhausted. Sometimes the baby is big and mom is small. It happens; fortunately, we have a few tricks up our sleeves to help our little ones find their way into their mother's arms.

Lacerations 101 (what it means if you tear)

We talked earlier about how episiotomies aren't routine anymore, because the majority of mothers can deliver the baby without damaging their vagina at all. We also learned that when mothers have an episiotomy, they sometimes have worse lacerations than they might have without one. Sometimes, though, mom's vaginal and perineal tissue (the area between the vagina and the rectum) can't stretch any farther, but she still needs to make a little more room for baby. That's when tears happen. As unpleasant (OK, terrifying) as that sounds, most tears are minor and easy to repair and heal up beautifully. Of course, it's far better if mom doesn't tear at all, and most providers use a variety of techniques (oil, warm compresses, perineal massage, and support) to prevent a tear from happening.

If a mom has abrasions or very minor lacerations that don't require stitching (we in the trade call those "skid marks")—she can expect to feel sore for a few days. If she tears or is one of the few who need an episiotomy, she'll need stitches to bring the tissues back together so they'll heal well. If mom has an epidural, she won't feel the stitching. If she doesn't, her doctor will give her a numbing injection of local anesthetic in the vaginal/perineal area before she starts the repair.

Tears and episiotomies are referred to in terms of degrees:

- **First-degree lacerations** involve only the skin around the vagina and perineum. This kind of tear may or may not need stitches and should heal very quickly. It may sting when you pee, but warm water, ice packs, and Lidocaine spray will help ease pain and promote healing.

- **Second-degree lacerations** involve the skin and muscle layer in the perineum. This definitely needs stitching and can be expected to be sore for about a week. Ice, warm water, Lidocaine spray, and anti-inflammatory medications should eliminate swelling and reduce pain.

- **Third-degree lacerations** involve the skin and perineal muscle layers plus the anal sphincter (the muscle that surrounds the anus and lets us squeeze it shut). Midwives usually consult with obstetricians for these kinds of repairs, which require extensive stitching and a custom-care approach to make sure mom heals correctly and doesn't have problems with bowel movements or sex later on. This kind of laceration can take months to heal completely.

- **Fourth-degree lacerations** go through the skin, vagina, perineum and rectum. This repair is often done in the operating room and always by an obstetrician. When repaired properly, these lacerations usually heal completely and don't cause mothers any long-lasting problems in terms of bowel movements or sex. If it's not done well (and in developing countries, where health care is limited, these childbirth injuries frequently go unrepaired), fourth-degree lacerations can cause incontinence, infection, and extreme disability.

No matter what shape your vagina, perineum, and vulva are in after you've given birth, avoiding constipation is super important. Even if you didn't have tearing or even skid marks, your lady parts have been through a lot. You do not want to have to strain to poop. Drink lots of water, eat fresh fruits and veggies, and take the stool softener your nurse offers you. Stool softeners are also available over the counter, so buy a bottle to keep at home, just in case.

I know what you're thinking: *If I tear, am I ever going to be normal down there again?* Yes, you will be. Midwives and doctors stitch up vaginas all day long, and they're really good at it. The vagina is resilient; it's designed to take a beating, and it's amazing at healing. It may take a few months before the soreness goes away enough for a vigorous romp, but you will heal and chances are extremely good that you will enjoy sex again.

Maybe this is TMI, but I had a great big laceration with my first baby and healed up so well I was pregnant again long before I planned to be. My midwife did an episiotomy with number two and I healed just fine in no time at all. No tearing at all with babies three and four. Did all this vaginal trauma ruin my sex life? Ummm . . . nope, not one little bit.

Body fluids, blood, and guts—all the gross stuff that happens during labor and why you shouldn't worry about it

If all pregnant women created a *Top Five Things I'm Dreading about Labor* list, most would include these three: fear of bleeding, fear of vomiting, and fear of pooping in front of people. Let me put your mind at ease—you have nothing to worry about. That's not because these three things don't ever happen—they do. They happen all the time. It's because bleeding, vomiting, and pooping in labor are so common that the people taking care of you won't bat an eye. Seriously—you can leak amniotic fluid off the side of your bed, poop while pushing, and totally miss the barf bowl, and it's no big deal to your nurse. We deal with body fluids all day long, and not only are we not shocked, offended, grossed out, or put out, but we're anticipating that you'll get messy. We'll go to the ends of the earth to help you feel clean, cared for, and relaxed about it. In fact, if your nurse has children, chances are good she barfed or pooped a bit during labor, too.

There's not much you can do about body fluids. It is just part of the many unpleasant indignities of labor and birth, and your nurses get that. We also understand that our patients haven't had anyone else attend to keeping their bottoms clean since they were in diapers, and we understand that can feel humiliating. That's why we're experts at this. We'll keep you stocked with disposable underwear and the biggest sanitary pads you've ever seen. We'll keep a basin or mini-bucket and a pile of washcloths handy, in case you need to throw up. We'll place dry

Chux (paper and plastic bed liners, aka puppy pads) and towels under your tush to keep you as dry as possible. If you're pushing and something extra comes out, we'll wipe you up before you even realize what happened. We're on it. I promise.

How about bleeding? This fear usually has less to do with embarrassment and more to do with basic mortality. There will be blood, probably quite a lot more than you expect, but in most cases the amount of blood you'll lose during labor and birth isn't dangerous. It may be messy, you may find it worrying, but in most cases it's not dangerous. When women do bleed too much, that's called hemorrhage, and we're on guard for that. We know that hemorrhage in childbirth is one of the leading causes of death for women in countries that lack medical care. Here in the United States, we're seeing increased cases of hemorrhage in relation to placental problems and too many C-sections. In most cases, however, if our patient is bleeding more than we like, we know what to do about it.

When women bleed excessive amounts *during labor*, we worry about the placenta separating from the uterine wall. This is called "placental abruption" (or placenta abruptio). Normally, the placenta doesn't separate until after the baby is born. If it separates before birth, this can be a straight up seriously scary emergency and you're going to the OR immediately. No messing around. Get that baby outta there, because without the placenta, your baby is in big, big trouble. Mom's in pretty big trouble too, because the placenta covers a large area inside the uterus that's rich with blood vessels (thus all the bleeding). Normally the uterus clamps down after the placenta is delivered, which reduces the surface area and diminishes bleeding. If the baby is still in the uterus when the placenta separates, the uterus can't clamp down, which means mom's going to bleed heavily. Sometimes only a bit of the placenta separates and mom and baby remain stable. Other times a large section separates; this is a C-section STAT situation.

Now that I've gone all scary on you, let me reassure you, this doesn't happen all that often. Here's what the National Institutes of Health[4] says:

Placental abruption, which includes any amount of placental separation before delivery, occurs in about 1 out of 150 deliveries. The severe form, which can cause the baby to die, occurs in only about 1 out of every 800 to 1,600 deliveries.

I like to take scary stats like that and flip them. When you turn those numbers around they read like this: In 149 out of 150 deliveries, the placenta does exactly what it's supposed to do and mother and baby are just fine. The severe form of placental abruption *does not happen* in greater than 99 percent of births. In other words, the odds that you'll experience this very rare emergency are *very* low.

Whether you're at home or in the hospital, you'll be the best person to gauge how much you're bleeding. How do you know whether your bleeding level is normal? Generally, if you're in labor and spotting or bleeding so little that you're not filling a pad quickly, you're probably fine. If you're filling a pad in an hour or less, your nurse, midwife, or doctor needs to check it out. If you're bleeding *and* have any of the following symptoms, get medical help right away—these may signal serious complications:

- Severe, nonstop abdominal or back pain
- A rigid abdomen that doesn't relax
- Contractions that are abnormally close together or don't relax at all
- Bright red blood

What if you're unsure whether you're having too much bleeding? Just hit the call button or call your provider. It's always smart to check in with your nurse, midwife, or doctor whenever you're worried. Don't even give it a second thought. We'd much rather check you out and tell you everything's OK than have you sit at home or in your hospital bed worrying—or, worse, have you call your bleeding to our attention too late for us to give you the care you might desperately need.

C-Sections, VBACs, and More

Currently, about one in three American women will deliver her baby by C-section. I'd like to see that number come way, way down, but until it does—and in case you have a C-section in your future—you'll need some solid information. Let's talk about how this surgery is performed, why it's become so common, and some alternatives that might help you avoid one if you'd prefer to.

You're scheduled for a C-section— what happens next?

Prescheduled, unscheduled, and emergency C-sections all go through the same basic procedures: surgery prep, anesthesia, surgery, birth, repair, recovery. Whatever the reason for having a C-section, most women feel anxious or frightened before surgery. It makes sense to wonder, "Is my baby going to be OK? And am I going to be OK?" It's major surgery, and even though we've minimized the significance and seriousness of this surgical procedure in recent years, it remains a pretty big deal.

Let's break down the basic processes involved in having a C-section so you'll feel less worried. Oh, and to answer those big questions—chances are excellent that both you and your baby are going to be OK. Obstetricians do this surgery all the time. They know what they're doing, and contrary to what many women think, it's usually not an emergency.

Presurgery

You'll need all this in place before you head to the operating room:

- Signed consent form indicating you understand the risks and benefits of having a C-section

- Dressed in a hospital gown (everything else off, including underwear, jewelry, bra, and so on)

- Fetal monitoring to determine baby's well-being

- Health history taken (make sure everybody knows your allergies, previous medical conditions, and surgeries)

- Verification that you haven't had anything to eat or drink recently. If you have eaten or had anything to drink, your C-section may have to be rescheduled.

- Vital signs evaluated (temperature, blood pressure, heart rate, respiratory rate, reflexes)

- IV started and fluids infusing

- Anesthesia consultation

- Pubic hair shaved or clipped in the area where an incision will be made

- OR clothing (scrubs) given to the one person accompanying you into the OR

Once all these are in place, you'll walk or be wheeled (in a chair or on your bed) into the operating room. Your partner will most likely be asked to wait a while before coming into the OR to be with you. That's because the rest of the prep procedures are done in a sterile environment that requires minimal distraction. Don't worry, he or she will be called into the OR before surgery starts.

In the OR

The anesthetist will meet you in the OR. The room will be cool and bright and you'll be offered heated blankets. You'll sit or lie on the edge of the operating bed (aka table) where the anesthetist will place cardiac and respiratory monitors on you and, if you don't already have one, will administer an epidural or spinal anesthesia (see Epidural 101, page 136). Your nurse will be right there with you, helping you to get in position and feel calm during this procedure. Her whole job is to be there for you. She knows you're nervous (the whole OR team knows), so don't hesitate to tell her if you need anything (a hug, a hand to hold, more blankets, a tissue, a moment—whatever you need). Once your anesthesia is done, you'll have a large grounding pad (sticky pad) applied to your thigh (it prevents electric cautery equipment from shocking you) and, if you don't already have one, a Foley (urinary) catheter will be inserted.

By this point, your legs will be numb. Don't worry about it. Your OR team will carefully move your body for you. Then you'll be assisted into a supine (lying on your back) position with a towel or blanket wedged under one hip to keep the weight of the uterus from compressing blood vessels that circulate blood to the uterus, placenta, and baby. Straps will be buckled around your legs to keep your body secure. Your arms will be placed on armrests. Some anesthetists place light Velcro straps on your arms, but many don't. If that feels restrictive to you, tell him you don't want them. Just be very careful you don't unintentionally reach into the sterile field (everything covered with blue paper). You'll be covered with a large paper and plastic blue paper drape that will be taped and clipped in place to prevent you from watching your own surgery and to make sure everything remains sterile. It also catches body fluids like amniotic fluid and blood.

The anesthetist and your doctor will test to make sure you can't feel any pain in your abdomen. You'll be fully conscious, and you may feel pressure and movement, and that's normal, but you shouldn't feel any pain. If you do, speak up loudly and your anesthetist will administer more medication. Once everyone is sure you're 100-percent comfortable, your partner will be escorted into the OR and seated at your side near your head, and surgery will begin.

Delivery

Surgery itself goes quickly. From the time your doctor makes the first incision (usually made horizontally near your bikini line and 4 to 5 inches long) to the time your baby is born will likely be 10 to 15 minutes. During that time you'll feel a bit of tugging, hear suction noises, and smell amniotic fluid and probably blood. You'll also hear your doctor and her assistant surgeon and techs talking. The anesthetist will be sitting at your head, and if you feel anything weird, he's there for you. You can talk to your partner, doctors, and nurses. You may feel queasy or you may feel perfectly fine. Pretty soon your doctor will say, "Here comes your baby," and voilà—your baby will be lifted from your belly. The time will be recorded, the sex will be announced, and your baby will be transferred to a team of nurses at a nearby radiant warmer. Your baby will be dried, quickly evaluated, and within just a few minutes handed to your partner at your side. You'll be able to touch your baby but probably won't be able to hold her until your surgery is over and you're transferred to your recovery bed.

Repair

The rest of your surgery will take anywhere from 20 to 40 minutes as your doctor delivers the placenta and sutures your uterus and muscle layers closed. She may use sutures (stitches), surgical staples, or surgical glue to close the skin layer. Then she'll push down firmly on your uterus to empty it of blood. You'll be cleaned up, bandaged, changed into a fresh gown (if necessary), and transferred to a gurney or recovery bed. You still won't be able to move, so your surgical team will do all the moving for you. Then you'll be tucked in with warm blankets and, as long as your baby is stable, she'll be snuggled into your arms.

Note: If your baby is experiencing complications, she'll most likely be transferred to the nursery for special care. Your partner has to make a hard choice at this point—stay with you or go to the nursery. If he decides to go to the nursery, he won't be allowed to return to the operating room but will be able to meet you in your recovery or postpartum room. You'll be able to visit your baby in the nursery as soon as you're stable, your anesthesia has worn off, and you can sit in a wheelchair (probably several hours after surgery).

Recovery

You'll be wheeled into the recovery room or your postpartum suite. If your baby has not been taken to the nursery for special care, she and your partner will go with you. Your nurse will take your vital signs and check your incision for bleeding frequently. She'll help you breast-feed and provide all your baby care. Your urinary catheter and IV will stay in place for approximately 12 to 24 hours or until you're able to get up and walk to the bathroom, drink fluids, and eat. You can probably take sips of water or suck on ice chips as soon as you're in the recovery room, but you probably won't be able to drink anything for a couple of hours or more. Some hospitals let you drink clear liquids and eat soft foods within several hours after surgery, but some make you wait quite a bit longer. That's because your digestion process will be drastically slowed down due to the trauma of surgery and administration of nar-cotic medication. Don't push it. You really don't want to throw up after surgery if you can avoid it. Nausea is common, and your nurse can give you antinausea medication in your IV. If you feel super hungry, ask for something to take the edge off, like Jell-O, juice, or broth. Once every-one's sure you're recovering well and aren't likely to throw up, they'll gradually advance your diet. You'll be eating normal foods within a day of surgery.

What about post-op pain? Your spinal or epidural anesthesia will wear off within a couple of hours after surgery, but you will probably have received a drug called Duramorph along with your anesthesia that will take most of your pain away for the first 12 to 24 hours. You will feel some pain, though, probably within a few hours of returning to your postpartum room. Don't let this pain get too severe. Ask for pain medica-tion as soon as you feel pain, and your nurse will give you IV or oral nar-cotics. This is important, because you'll be expected to get up out of bed within a matter of hours after surgery. You'll need your pain medications to enable you to move around. This is no time to be stoic and avoid pain medications. This is the time to take them. Seriously—just take them.

That's what you can expect from a C-section. You'll feel better day by day; within 12 to 24 hours you'll be able to walk to and from the bathroom, your baby's crib, and maybe the couch, and you'll go home from the hospital in 3 or 4 days. You'll be tired, sore, and unable to do much for at least the first week or two, but each day should get easier. Keep in mind that you'll also be breastfeeding or bottle feeding and waking up at night to feed your baby, so expect to feel exhausted. Make sure you have lots of extra hands on deck for at least the first couple of weeks. There's no way you can manage recovering from major abdominal surgery plus take full responsibility for your baby any sooner than that. By week 3, most women are able to take full charge, though they shouldn't be expected to work at full capacity. By 6 weeks out, most women are considered fully recovered, though if we're going to be real about it, most don't feel 100 percent recovered for quite a while longer. It's major surgery. Let your body have all the time it needs to heal and adjust to life with a new baby.

You want a vaginal birth after cesarean (VBAC)—how can you have one, and what are the risks?

If a previous pregnancy ended with a C-section, your next one might, too. That's because in the American birth industry, the rigid policy of *once a C-section, always a C-section* is still entrenched in many parts of the country where vaginal birth after cesarean (VBAC) bans can be darn near impossible to get around. That's not because C-sections are always the safest birth option for women who've had previous C-sections. They're not. Most of the time VBAC is the safer choice.

What's the problem with VBACs? In fewer than 1 percent of all VBACs attempted, the pressure of contractions can cause the uterine scar (created by the first C-section) to rupture, which could result in massive hemorrhage and potentially the death of mother and baby. That's a frightening and serious situation, so it's a valid concern. In an attempt to prevent that 1-percent tragedy from occurring, doctors and hospitals required 100 percent of mothers with a prior C-section to forgo VBAC and undergo repeat C-sections. The problem is, C-sections can also cause massive hemorrhage, infection, and the death of mother and baby. It's largely because of VBAC bans that we now have the highest C-section rate we've ever had and our maternal mortality and morbidity rates are higher than they've been in decades and continue to climb.

How did things come to this? In 1965, the C-section rate was only 4.5 percent, but women who had one had subsequent babies via C-section, too. By 1981, C-sections had become the go-to solution for many obstetric complications, and the C-section rate rose to 17.9 percent. By 1985 it was 22.7 percent, and half of those surgeries were done simply because the mother had a previous C-section.

As the C-section rate continued to climb, evidence mounted that doing so many surgeries was causing harm instead of preventing it. The National Institutes of Health (NIH) stepped in, instigating a panel to question the necessity of routine repeat C-sections and VBAC bans. Careful studies determined that the risks from repeat C-sections were higher than those associated with VBAC, and eventually the NIH and the American Congress of Obstetricians and Gynecologists (ACOG) relaxed the ban and created new standards. Throughout the 1980s and early 1990s VBAC rates increased, and many doctors encouraged their patients to give it a try.

However, two studies, in 1996 and 2001, indicated that VBAC risks were significantly higher than those associated with repeat C-sections. While questions, controversy, and criticism surrounded these studies' conclusions, their opinions were enough for insurance providers to sound an alarm and for ACOG to dramatically change the criteria under which women could attempt VBACs. Insurance companies refused to cover hospitals for VBACs unless a surgeon and an anesthetist were on the hospital unit throughout active labor for any woman attempting VBAC. Doctors and hospitals didn't want to assume that much risk of a lawsuit, and most instigated strict VBAC bans.

Things got ugly when women who didn't want surgery or didn't think they needed it couldn't find a hospital or provider willing to do VBAC. Some women even faced a threat of imprisonment or loss of newborn custody if they refused surgery. Many women considered these VBAC bans a human rights violation, denying them their right to decide what would or would not happen to their bodies. Unnecessary surgeries were forced on women, even as new data showed that VBAC bans and unnecessary repeat C-sections were dangerous and even deadly. As the C-section rate continued to rise, so did U.S. maternal mortality and morbidity rates. Women suffered severe complications, either directly from surgery or from uterine scarring during subsequent pregnancies. Placentas attached abnormally to scarred uteruses, causing women to bleed profusely. Postsurgical infections became more common and increasingly difficult to treat. Babies wound up in the NICU at alarming rates, with infections, breathing problems, and complications associated with prematurity because repeat C-sections were often scheduled a couple of weeks before a mother's due date.

In 2009 the NIH stepped in again and called for a review of maternal and newborn health statistics related to C-sections and VBACs. This forced ACOG to review its practices and in 2010 to revise its policies once again. In 2010, ACOG issued this statement: "Approximately 60–80 percent of appropriate candidates who attempt VBAC will be successful. A VBAC avoids major abdominal surgery, lowers a woman's risk of hemorrhage and infection, and shortens postpartum recovery. It may also help women avoid the possible future risks of having multiple cesareans such as hysterectomy, bowel and bladder injury, transfusion, infection, and abnormal placental conditions (placenta previa and placenta accreta)."[1]

What happens to the 20 to 40 percent who aren't successful? They'll have a C-section, but that's a more appropriate use of surgery than forcing 100 percent of women seeking a VBAC to have one they probably don't need.

Where does that leave us today? Even though VBAC bans have been lifted, many doctors and hospitals remain dug in and won't allow it. What are women's options then? Some women can shop around in their community for doctors and midwives who support VBAC. But for women who live in small towns and rural areas, there are no practical solutions other than traveling long distances to seek care in a VBAC-supportive hospital.

For many women, their only choice has been to either have a surgery they don't need or have a home birth or deliver at an out-of-hospital birth center. I worry about this, since the outcome of being in that less-than-1-percent group that suffers a uterine rupture is dire. The only way to survive this life-threatening emergency is immediate surgical intervention and access to a blood bank and NICU. Fortunately, hospitals are waking up to their role in forcing women into the health care margins.

If you want a VBAC but your doctor is reluctant, ask him why he thinks another C-section is your best health care option. It might be because of the way your previous surgical incision was made. If you had a vertical uterine incision (running down the length of your uterus rather than across it) instead of the more standard low, horizontal one, that puts you at increased risk for rupture. If you're carrying twins or an unusually big baby, many doctors feel that's too much risk, even though studies don't support that opinion. If he says it's because you have a weird placenta or it's covering your cervix, or your baby's in a transverse (sideways) position, or some other legit medical indication, then it sounds like he has valid reasons for recommending another C-section. If he says it's because he never does VBACs, tell him he's too old-school for you, and start shopping around.

You have twins or your baby is breech— can you still have a vaginal birth?

The pendulum has swung back and forth so many times regarding when women can or can't deliver babies vaginally. For thousands of years, women delivered breech (when the baby is in a position other than head down) and multiple babies vaginally, and most survived. There weren't any other options, so midwives learned techniques for delivering these challenging babies. Even as recently as the 1980s and 1990s, twins and certain breech babies were routinely delivered vaginally. There were certain qualifying conditions, of course; for instance, twin A (the one closest to the vagina) had to be head down. Breech babies had to be in a frank breech position (butt near the vagina, legs straight up in front of the body) and full term. But sometime in the 1990s, the climate for vaginal deliveries changed so that all twins and breeches were routinely delivered by scheduled C-section.

Nowadays, most doctors continue to deliver these babies by C-section, primarily because that's how they were trained, but also because they believe it's the least risky way to go. Breech babies can present specific complications like a prolapsed umbilical cord (which falls into the vagina before the rest of the body, which can cause baby's blood supply to be compressed) or the head getting stuck after the body has been delivered. It's issues like these that prevent many doctors from delivering twins vaginally. If twin A is head down but twin B is breech, they worry that even if the first baby is born vaginally, the second one might not move into a good birthing position. Therefore, most doctors won't even attempt a vaginal delivery even when both babies are in a good birthing position. However, recent studies indicate there's no benefit to routinely doing a C-section for twins, and every surgery puts mom and babies at increased risk for other complications.

If mom is carrying triplets, having a C-section is still considered the safest way to deliver. That's a lot of umbilical cords, bodies, arms, and legs to manage delivering safely through the birth canal. Most doctors feel most capable of achieving safe births of multiples via C-section.

What if your baby is breech and you want a vaginal birth? If your due date is still several week away, chances are excellent that your baby will move into a head-down (cephalic) position on his own. There are several things you can do to nudge him in that direction.

The Webster technique is a series of chiropractic adjustments that help balance pelvic muscles so baby can move into a cephalic position. Some studies say this technique is successful 82 percent of the time.[2] If your chiropractor is experienced taking care of pregnant women and knows how to do the procedure, this procedure is safe and definitely worth a try.

Moxibustion is done by acupuncturists who apply heat to specific acupuncture points to stimulate fetal activity. Varying studies claim success rates between 30 and 80 percent.[3] This is a noninvasive procedure with no side effects and definitely worth a try. Should you tell your doctor you're seeing an acupuncturist? Why not? She may think it's a waste of time or too "alternative" for her tastes, but so what? A 30- to 80-percent success rate speaks for itself.

The Tilt is a maneuver you can do on your own. Lie on your back with your feet on a chair or the couch and your hips elevated about $1^1/_2$ feet above your head and supported with several pillows under your butt for several 15- to 20-minute sessions per day. This gives baby room to wiggle into a head-down position. If you're seeing a midwife, she may suggest you try this procedure. If you're seeing a doctor, that's not likely—not because the procedure is dangerous or ineffective, but because doctors are usually more into medical interventions than alternative ones. Still, this is fairly easy to do and just might work.

If these techniques don't work, doctors and midwives can attempt a technique called an "external cephalic version." This is done in the hospital because if the baby doesn't tolerate the procedure well (which happens occasionally), there's immediate access to emergency care. A "version" is a technique in which the doctor or midwife repositions baby by pressing down on mom's abdomen in a way that encourages baby to reposition herself into a head-down position. It may require that mom receive a medication to relax her abdominal muscles and uterus. Sometimes mom is given an epidural prior to having a version. Sometimes this is followed by an immediate induction, to facilitate a delivery before baby can flip back into a breech position. Sometimes mom is wrapped in an abdominal binder (sort of like a wide stretchy corset) to prevent baby from flipping back.

If your breech baby doesn't flip or you have twins and you want a vaginal birth, make sure your midwife or doctor has experience and knows how to accomplish it. Talk to your providers well in advance of delivery and find out if they've been trained and had experience and success and if they're comfortable giving a vaginal birth a try. Each of these requires a specific skill set, but considering the very established C-section culture that many doctors and midwives have worked and trained in lately, it's a skill set many don't have. Not that many midwives feel really comfortable managing breech and twin vaginal births.

It's easy to assume that if doctors are nervous about doing these alternative births vaginally, then it must be because they're inherently dangerous. That's not always the case. An awful lot of the time twin and breech vaginal births are entirely safe for mom and baby. Some cases call for delivery by C-section, but we don't need to deliver 100 percent of breech and twin babies by C-section just because a few need to be. It's not like C-sections are a risk-free proposition, y'know.

CHAPTER 13

Once the Baby Is Born

Delivering your baby is just the beginning. A lot happens in the hours and days that follow birth. Here's a rundown of some common and not-so-common tests, treatments, and scenarios you and your baby might encounter.

How to decide which tests and shots your baby will get in the delivery room and nursery

If you deliver your baby in a traditional maternity unit, you want to be very clear with your doctor, midwife, and nurses about what happens to your baby immediately after delivery. If your baby is healthy, then the best-case scenario has your newborn transferring directly after birth to your abdomen or chest—skin-to-skin in all her wet, slippery glory. Her cord can be left unclamped until it stops pulsing, or longer, to ensure she gets all the blood that's left in the cord and placenta after birth.

If she's born by C-section, that's (probably) not going to happen. Instead, she'll exit your abdomen, the cord will be immediately clamped and cut, and she'll be transferred to a nearby radiant warmer where nurses will evaluate her, take her vital signs, dry her off, and, if she's healthy, wrap her in blankets before she's transferred to your partner's waiting arms. If she's showing signs of illness or needs special care, she'll likely go to the nursery shortly after birth, where she'll receive extra medical attention.

But let's assume she's healthy and stable and can therefore stay with you right after birth. As soon as she's born, your nurse or midwife will listen to your baby's heart and breathing. She'll dry your baby off so she doesn't lose excess body heat. Her Apgar scores for muscle tone, cry, color, respirations, and activity will be evaluated and recorded. Her vitals and temperature will be checked at frequent intervals. If your baby is skin-to-skin with you, these evaluative procedures can be done in your arms. This is the ideal situation—leave mom and baby together as much as possible to optimize bonding and make baby's transition to the world as smooth and cuddly as possible.

In some hospitals, though, the cord is immediately clamped and cut (often by dad) and baby is transferred to a nearby radiant warmer. All the initial evaluative procedures are done before mom has a chance to get her hands on her baby. This isn't necessary in most cases (it's just that hospital's routine), and if your nurses are told in advance that you prefer to have baby stay with you, they should be happy to accommodate you. If your hospital is particularly rigid about procedures or they're worried about your baby or you're exhausted or having complications, then baby goes to the warmer.

It's not uncommon for nurses to try and get as many newborn care procedures out of the way as possible while they have baby on the warmer. This might include giving baby shots and blood tests in addition to doing Apgar scores, drying, and evaluation. Maybe this is no big deal to you, but I think that's a pretty harsh welcome for your baby. If your baby doesn't need special care, I recommend you tell the staff to wait on all that until you and your baby have had time together. A healthy baby doesn't need shots and blood tests so soon after birth.

Why do nurses do all those procedures immediately if they're not absolutely necessary? Because we have a very long list of tasks to complete with mom and baby within a very short period of time after birth, before we take on our next patient or turn our mother-baby couplet over to the next nurse. Nurses have to be experts at multitasking, and if we can take baby's vitals, do a vaccination and vitamin K shot, put antibiotics in eyes, slap on a diaper, and put identification bands on baby's arm and leg in the time it takes the doctor to deliver the placenta and stitch up a perineum—well then, that's considered being a good nurse. Although that's the reality of nursing in many maternity units, I think being a good nurse should really be about making sure mother and baby have the best possible start in life, and frankly, that usually doesn't have to include needles and tests and separation from mom.

Here are the routine delivery room tests and shots done on normal healthy babies that may done immediately but can totally be delayed or administered in mom's arms.

Umbilical cord is clamped and cut

There's a growing realization that the umbilical cord and placenta contain a significant volume of blood that baby needs. In most hospital-based deliveries the cord is clamped immediately after birth. That shuts off the flow of blood from the placenta to baby. The remaining blood volume left in the cord and placenta flows into a basin and gets thrown out. If cord clamping is delayed, though, then all that cord/placenta blood volume can transfer to baby, which increases her circulating blood volume significantly. Imagine how you'd feel if you were trying to transition to life without full access to your allotted blood volume. You'd feel weak, disoriented, and downright puny. The World Health Organization now recommends that the umbilical cord *not* be cut immediately after birth (this is called "delayed cord clamping"), and providers are being trained to wait at least 1 to 3 minutes after birth before clamping. The WHO says that allowing blood to flow to the newborn can help prevent anemia.

Identification bands placed on baby's arms and legs and parents' arms

This should be done ASAP after birth, because if baby needs to be taken out of mom's room to the nursery, ID bands with matching numbers are our best way of guaranteeing that babies aren't switched.

Antibiotic cream in baby's eyes

The drug of choice used on almost all newborns here in the United States is erythromycin cream, which goes in baby's eyes ASAP after birth. Its original function was to treat gonorrhea infection from causing blindness, but it also acts to prevent newborn eye infections caused by bacteria picked up during the birth process. While erythromycin cream does not hurt, it does make baby's vision blurry because it creates a temporary film on baby's eyes.

Vitamin K injection

This vitamin shot is given to virtually all babies to prevent a condition called hemorrhagic disease of the newborn, which is said to affect between 0.001 and 1.5 percent of all babies born.[1] This condition is also called vitamin K deficiency bleeding, which means the baby doesn't have enough vitamin K to clot blood. Birth can cause significant bruising to babies, and if they have this condition, and their blood doesn't clot, they could potentially have very significant internal bleeding. Since we don't know in advance which babies have this rare disorder, we give all newborns a vitamin K shot ASAP after birth. It is possible to give this vitamin orally, but it requires several doses given over a very long period of time (weeks to months) to achieve the same effect as one injection.

Hepatitis B vaccination

Parents have to sign a consent form in advance before their baby receives this shot. Since this consent is often lumped in with lots of other admitting paperwork, many parents don't realize they can opt out. Hepatitis B is a liver disease that results from infection with the hepatitis B virus due to contact with blood, semen, and other body fluids of an infected person. This vaccine is often administered shortly after birth because it's given in three doses spread out over several months. Pediatricians and public health officials figure that if they can get most newborns vaccinated before they leave the hospital, then if the parents don't bring baby back in for further pediatric care, they will have received at least one of the three doses, and that may provide partial protection. Essentially, hep B is contracted through sex or shared needle use. Presumably, your baby is not going to be engaging in either of those activities, so you can definitely postpone this shot without worrying your baby will be at risk. There will be plenty of time later for your baby to get all three shots and be fully protected against hepatitis B. If your pediatrician is adamant that your baby needs this vaccination ASAP, ask why and what the risks are if you wait, and make sure you communicate your reasons why you might want to wait.

Glucose test

If baby is showing signs of having low glucose (low body temperature, shaky or jittery muscle movements, lethargy), a blood test may be done by poking his heel to check his blood sugar level. Glucose is essential for keeping the brain and vital organs fed and functioning. If baby is working hard to keep himself warm or to breathe, he may quickly use up the glucose he had stored in his blood. If baby is breastfed shortly after birth, though, and kept warm through skin-to-skin contact or a radiant warmer or dry blankets, his glucose level should be just fine. Some hospitals do this test on all babies, though it's necessary on only a few. Tell your nurses and care providers that you want to be informed what tests they'll be performing on your baby *before* they're done and why they're doing them. That gives you the opportunity to discuss and understand risks and benefits and to participate in a decision about whether or not your baby really needs "routine" testing.

Routine vital signs

Baby's temperature, heart, and respiratory rate will be evaluated frequently to make sure baby is warm, stable, and not having trouble breathing and that she's making the transition to life outside the uterus smoothly. Vital signs can be taken in mom's arms as easily as anywhere.

Apgar scores

This test is done through visual observation when baby is 1 minute and 5 minutes old. We look at five categories (breathing, heart rate, muscle tone, reflexes, and skin color) and each gets scored with a 0, 1, or 2 depending on how baby appears. An Apgar score of 9/10 means baby's doing great at 1 minute and perfectly at 5 minutes. Almost no baby gets a score of 10 at 1 minute. They just need a little time to adjust. This test can be done in mom's arms.

Weight and measurement

Baby will be placed on a scale to determine her birth weight. Then she'll be measured from head to toe and around the circumference of her head. As eager as most parents are to know how big their baby is (and some parents ask the weight before baby's even left their midwife's hands), the baby will weigh essentially the same at one hour as she does immediately after birth.

Footprints

Baby's feet will be pressed onto an inkpad and then onto a hospital birth certificate (not a legal document) as a memento of baby's birth. It's a tradition, not a medical necessity, but one most of us treasure. I've had fathers request we use another inkpad to press the footprints onto his arm or back too (some even use this as a stencil for a tattoo). A few hospitals still try to do handprints, but babies like to keep their tiny fists clenched, which doesn't make for great prints. This is usually done right before a bath.

Baby bath

Most nurses will wait until baby is at least a couple of hours old before giving her a bath. Some parents ask that baby be bathed immediately, but we want to make sure baby is stable and warm before we do anything as stimulating as a bath. If the blood and goop most babies have on their skin immediately after birth bothers you, no worries; your nurse can dry your baby off with heated blankets. The bath may happen in the sink, in a portable tub, or as a sponge bath in the baby's warmer. Both parents will be invited to observe, and this first bath is used as a teaching moment so first-time parents begin to learn how to handle and care for their baby.

Breastfeeding

In a perfect world, all babies would be encouraged to nurse ASAP after birth. Lots of babies will do just that, especially when they're skin-to-skin with mom. However, plenty of babies need some time to chill out before they get down to the work of nursing. Birth is rough on babies, and while some will instinctively go for the comfort of the breast, others need a little time to simply adjust to their new existence. All healthy babies should be given immediate access to the breast, but don't worry if yours doesn't latch on right away. He'll get around to it when he's ready.

When your baby needs intensive care

Most babies are born healthy, well, and ready to meet life head-on. Some, however, need extra help because they are premature, are having trouble breathing, have had a traumatic birth, or have an illness or injury. If your health care team suspects trouble in advance, they'll have extra personnel present at birth to make sure all of baby's needs are met. If baby's poor health comes as a surprise, your delivery room team knows what to do. In addition to being trained in advanced emergency life support procedures, they know how to get extra nurses, a pediatrician, respiratory support—whoever they need—STAT!

Sometimes, all baby needs is a few minutes, a little oxygen, some extra fluids, or a little suctioning and he snaps out of his post-birth funk. Other times, though, a baby needs to go to the neonatal intensive care unit (NICU) as quickly as possible so experts can evaluate what he needs and how to treat him. There's no time for snuggling skin-to-skin with mom or breastfeeding immediately after birth. This is understandably hard on parents, but it's for their baby's well-being.

If mom has just delivered, she most likely will not be stable enough to go to the NICU with baby. However, the baby's other parent or another family member can often accompany baby and the medical team. In some circumstances—if the nursery is crowded, if baby's parent is sick, or if baby is in deep trouble—the medical team may ask the parent to wait outside the nursery. This is not an attempt to exclude them. It's an attempt to protect the other babies or to focus 100 percent of their attention and resources on the baby. More often, though, the parent is brought into the nursery and one nurse acts as his point person to keep him informed of all the procedures being done to evaluate and treat their baby.

Baby will be placed under a radiant warmer, which keeps him warm while also allowing the NICU team to surround him on three sides and observe his skin color, breathing, and behavior. The priorities of NICU care are the ABC's: airway, breathing, and circulation. Baby's airway will be evaluated to make sure it's open and able to take in air. If it's blocked, it will be suctioned and, if necessary, supported with an artificial airway (a molded plastic tube placed in baby's mouth and throat). Breathing will be evaluated with monitor stickers and leads and by stethoscope and visual assessment. Baby's blood oxygen level will be assessed with a pulse oximeter through a monitor taped to his foot. If he needs oxygen, it will be delivered through a mask placed over his nose and mouth, or through a nasal cannula (a small plastic tube that goes into the nose) or by oxygen tent (a clear plastic device that's placed over baby's head and has oxygen pumped in). Circulation is assessed through sticker monitors placed on baby's chest attached to wires. These wires do not deliver electricity to baby; they deliver information from baby to a computerized machine that lets staff know how often his heart is beating. They'll check his blood pressure with the teensiest blood pressure cuff you've ever seen.

Your baby may get a chest X-ray to look for pneumonia or problems with his lungs. He will have blood drawn from his foot or through a vein in the back of the hand, foot, inside the elbow, or on his head. This blood will be sent to the lab and checked for infection, anemia, glucose level, and whatever else the pediatrician orders. An IV will be started almost immediately, and sometimes blood can be drawn from the IV to save baby an extra poke. The IV will be baby's access line for fluids and medications. The medications baby receives will be determined by the pediatrician's diagnosis.

How will baby be fed? At first, when baby is being admitted and evaluated, baby won't be fed. He may receive glucose by IV to keep his blood sugar stable, but he probably won't be able to breastfeed. Sick babies don't usually have enough energy. Once he's stabilized, and depending on what condition landed him in the NICU, he may be able to be breastfed or receive mom's pumped breast milk.

Baby's course of treatment in the NICU varies depending on what's wrong with him. Mom will be able to come to the NICU to visit as soon as she's recovered from birth. Some babies recover quickly and are able to go back to mom's room; others need more time in the nursery, where nurses can keep their eyes on him around the clock. Some very sick babies will even spend weeks to months in the nursery. NICU nurses know this is terribly hard on parents, and they usually go to great lengths to make the nursery the very best first home they can for baby.

For all the wires, monitors, tubes, alarms, and IVs that are all over the NICU, there's a calm, coordinated kind of organization amid what looks to most parents like chaos. It's part of the NICU's job to incorporate parents into their routines, to teach them how to care for their compromised baby, and to prepare them to eventually take their baby home. Take the time you need to adjust to your new normal and the shock of not having a healthy baby in your arms, then jump in. Ask questions, talk to the nurses, make your wishes known, and do as much baby care as your baby is capable of receiving. As weird a place as a NICU is, it's important to remember that it's your nursery, too. Even more important to remember is that it's your baby, not theirs. But also remember this—the medical team that works in the NICU is expert at saving babies' lives, and save them they do. It's amazing what these miracle workers can do, and chances are very, very good they'll work miracles for your baby, too.

CHAPTER 14

Processing and Healing Postpartum

You did it. You made it through pregnancy and delivered your baby, and now you're a mother. You are parents. You have a new family or a bigger family. Go you! Now what?

The postpartum period is sometimes referred to as the fourth trimester, as your body transitions from baby-making to milk-making. Your hormones switch gears yet again as your uterus shrinks and heals and your breasts take on a brand-new function. Your mental acuity shifts to include your new responsibility for the life of a completely vulnerable newborn. You take on and adjust to your new identity—no longer just yourself, but now somebody's mother. And you do all that on very little, broken sleep, with a sore butt or belly and leaky boobs.

In this section we'll talk about what's normal, what's not, and what's somewhere in between. It's important to remember that the way you feel during the next few months is not how you should expect to feel forever. This is not your new state of being. It's an altered state known as "being postpartum." Some parents soar through this stage of life and some don't. Let's talk about that.

Processing your birth experience

Most women spend their prepregnancy lives comparing and contrasting what they think their pregnancy will be like against their sisters' and friends' experiences. When they finally go through it themselves, the real thing is almost never exactly what they'd expected.

Perhaps your first labor was a lot harder than you thought it would be. Or maybe you're among the few who thought it was a breeze. Maybe your birth philosophy categorized labor as intense rather than painful, but you hadn't fully realized just how intense it would be. Maybe you envisioned yourself as a Zen beauty, all deep breathing and golden light, and instead you shrieked expletives like a pack of teenage boys. Maybe you thought you'd be screaming and yelling, and instead, you turned inward, relaxing into each contraction in silence. Maybe you thought your partner would faint and were surprised to find that he or she was tender and helpful. Maybe you anticipated a perfect birth, and instead you were among the 15 percent who had serious complications. Whatever your experience, if this was your first birth, I'd bet it wasn't entirely like you thought it would be.

If this was your second birth, I bet this was the birth you thought you'd have when you created your birth plan for baby number one. I bet your body responded more smoothly and you were able to work with each contraction more efficiently. Labor and pushing went faster, recovery is going more smoothly, and the whole experience has been a lot saner and more under control. If it was your third or fourth child, you knew exactly what to expect but left room to be caught by surprise. While every labor and birth goes through the same processes (even when it's a C-section), each one is unique, because even with an experienced mother, every baby is a brand-new experience.

Some women have a hard time reconciling the reality of their birth with what they'd anticipated. They create a thoughtful birth plan, and when their reality doesn't line up with what they'd anticipated, they feel a confusing tangle of emotions. Some feel betrayed by the medical system or staff, or they feel like a wimp because they got an epidural when they intended to go natural. Others are stunned they had a C-section or question whether they really needed one. Some women feel like they've been sold a bill of goods by women who said they could do it without drugs; others feel like the epidural they always planned on wasn't the piece o' cake they'd heard it would be.

Birth is like that—unpredictable. It's physical, spiritual, emotional, intellectual, painful, joyful, athletic, exhausting, intense, peaceful, frightening, empowering—it's everything. Prepare all you want, but there's no way your brain can wrap itself around an experience like that in advance.

For some women, the gap between their expectation and reality is so wide, they're unable to make the emotional leap. Add on sleep deprivation and hormonal chaos, and they plunge into such deep emotional waters that they sink into depression. If they're well supported, they'll be able to access the help they need to create a bridge to healthy motherhood. If not, well, we all know women who suffer with postpartum depression. It's more common than we think.

So how do we begin to process the experience? I think an honest debriefing session should be part of every birth. I think women should have scheduled time to sit with their midwives or doctors and nurses to talk through what happened and their feelings about it all. Since that type of formal conversation isn't scheduled into most postpartum experiences, perhaps the best thing we can do is create our own debriefing sessions. We can invite our providers to talk it through with us, or we can talk it out with our mother, sisters, friends, and family. We can create space to discuss what birth is really like for women. We can talk about the good, the bad, and the ugly, the unexpected happiness, trauma, exhaustion, and elation. We can share our stories honestly, openly, and without judgment, putting our births in perspective.

What if you know you're not bridging the gap well? If you're experiencing unremitting anger, sadness, depression, or what many mothers report—a feeling of "nothingness," neither happiness nor sadness, but a deep sense of blah—you may need more support than your partner or family can provide. Tell your midwife or doctor. You may simply be suffering from deep fatigue, but you may also be experiencing depression. Either way, you need help. That might mean extra nighttime help, a therapist, a prescription, or an extra week with your mom nearby. Whatever you need to get through this huge life transition, you deserve it. Don't hesitate to ask for what you need.

For decades now American women have been expected to hop off the delivery bed and back into their prepregnancy selves with little or no recovery time. Unlike in other cultures, which designate the first month after birth as a time when mom is expected to do nothing more than feed her baby and rest, American mothers are given a day or two in the hospital, maybe another week of rest at home, and then they'd better get a move on. By 6 weeks postpartum we expect most mothers to be back at work and able to juggle it all. Fortunately, people are now getting the message that women cannot be expected to snap back from birth and into the role of motherhood without serious support, rest, and time. We haven't changed enough about the culture of motherhood yet to prevent mothers from experiencing anxiety and depression, but word is getting out. Unfortunately, it's taken a host of women with postpartum depression to send the message.

What can you do to reconcile your birth plans with your birth reality? Give yourself time. Recognize that you didn't really know what to plan for. Know that you're in good company, because it's like this for most mothers. Then ask for help and be willing to receive it. You'll have a lifetime of being your child's mother. You don't have to do it at 100-percent capacity right away. Give yourself a break.

Healing, bleeding, leaking, and cramps— what's normal, what's not?

Just when you thought all the discomfort and indignities of pregnancy, labor, and birth were over, may we introduce the postpartum period? It's 4 to 6 weeks (more or less) with a sore vagina and/or belly, persistent bleeding and cramps, and breasts that swell, fill with milk, leak, squirt, ache, sting, crack, and bruise. All that while sleeping (or not) in 2-hour increments.

If you had a vaginal birth, even if you didn't have a tear, laceration, or episiotomy, you're probably going to feel swollen and sore for the first few days to a week after delivery. Soaking in a warm tub feels great, and ice packs help a lot. So do ibuprofen, Vicodin, and Lidocaine spray (available over the counter at your drugstore). Here's a handy tip: Stock up on the biggest feminine hygiene pads you can find (overnighters). Pour water over a few and stick them in the freezer. Slide one into your underwear for 15 minutes a few times per day to reduce inflammation and reduce pain. You might want to put a towel or Chux under your tush in case it thaws.

If you had a vaginal laceration and repair, you have stitches (aka sutures). Your biggest priorities are to (1) avoid constipation so you don't put stress on the sutures and (2) keep this area clean. Use a squirt bottle to clean up every time you use the bathroom, and change your pads frequently. If you notice any foul odor, increased pain, bleeding, or any other kind of drainage coming from your vagina, call your midwife or doctor. You may have an infection. Most women heal very well, and while they may still feel achy, by their 6-week postpartum appointment, their vagina should be almost back to normal.

If you've had a C-section, your incision will feel pretty sore for the first week. You'll be prescribed pain pills (Vicodin, oxycodone) and ibuprofen. Take them. There are no prizes for biting a bullet and going med-free, and if you don't manage your pain, you'll avoid getting up and around as soon as you should. Also, drink lots of fluids, eat plenty of fruits and veggies, and take a stool softener, because narcotic pain meds cause constipation. Get up and walk. Of course you'll be picking up your baby, but don't lift anything heavier for the first week. No housework, exercise, or driving until you're off the pain pills and have your energy back *and* your doc says it's OK. By the time you reach your 6-week checkup, you should be feeling pretty darn well.

Some women are concerned that taking pain pills will ruin their breast milk. Don't worry too much about that. What little bit may transfer into your milk during the few days to a week or more isn't enough to cause any problems. Millions of women take narcotic pain pills for the first week or so after their births, and their babies are just fine. Take your medications as prescribed when you need them and switch to non-narcotic drugs as your pain level diminishes. If you still have so much pain within a week or so after delivery that you need narcotics in order to function, make sure your doctor or midwife knows. They can help evaluate your ongoing pain, determine which medications are most appropriate while breastfeeding, and help you get back on your feet. When mothers take narcotics for too long they risk becoming dependent or addicted and their babies might risk adverse effects associated with long-term exposure.

You'll have cramps, much like a period, for the first few days after delivery. Your uterus is tightening up to reduce its internal surface area where the placenta separated and to empty out all the remnants from your pregnancy. Many women have cramps when they breastfeed, too, since breastfeeding stimulates a release of oxytocin (the hormone that causes contractions). Ibuprofen, heat, baths, rest, and pain pills will make you feel a whole lot better.

What about that bleeding? Some women think that if they have a C-section they won't have postpartum bleeding. Wrong. Every new mother has vaginal bleeding. Some have more than others, but for most women the first few days will be like a heavy period. Small clots are common (smaller than a grape), but large clots aren't normal; if you pass any, you should contact your nurse, midwife, or doctor. The bleeding should taper off and gradually become lighter day by day. If you have a sudden increase in bleeding or after the first few days you have a return of bright red blood, that's a sign you're doing too much. Your uterus is doing its best to clamp down and return to its prepregnancy size, but you have to do your part with lots of rest.

After the first week or so, your bleeding will be much like the lightest days of your period, but one that lasts for a month. It's not uncommon to have spotting for up to 6 weeks after delivery. After that, you might not have a period again for quite some time, especially if you're breastfeeding. Some women, though, start right back into a normal menstrual cycle within a month or two of birth.

We'll tackle how to manage your breasts in Chapter 16, but while you're out shopping for huge sanitary napkins, hop over to the aisle that sells nursing pads, because the girls are gonna leak.

Nobody thinks the postpartum period is a glamorous time of life. After all you've been through, I really think women should be given (1) a reprieve from leaking, bleeding, and cramping and (2) a huge dose of instant healing. Apparently, though, Mother Nature has another plan, which includes all kinds of messiness and unpleasantness designed to keep new mothers at home, in bed, and snuggling with their newborn. Maybe she knows what she's doing.

Will you ever be normal down there again?

Yes, you will. There. Feel better?

In a perfect birth, the baby slides right out and everything goes back to the way it was pre-baby in no time at all. More often, even when a midwife or doctor provides excellent perineal support and mom is a smooth pusher, the vagina, vulva, and perineum experience some minor to major irritation, laceration, and edema—about what you'd expect from pushing a big ol' baby through a relatively tight space.

Don't let the way your vulvar area looks and feels in the days and weeks after birth be your measure for whether or not you'll ever be back to normal. Things can look far from normal for a while, even if you didn't have any tears or lacerations. Most women swell a bit after birth. Some women have so much swelling it looks frightening. Bruising is normal. So are sutures, if you had a tear or episiotomy. In very rare cases, moms develop a hematoma—a blood-filled pocket underneath the skin. Don't worry. Wait a month, and see how much you've healed. It's amazing how fast women heal when they've had good care at birth and they're given ample opportunities to rest. Continue using ice packs for as long as you notice swelling. Soak in a tub a few times a day to relieve soreness and promote healing (safe, even with stitches) and pretty soon you'll feel and look more like yourself. You may not feel 100 percent back to normal by the time you reach your 6-week postpartum checkup, but give it time. For the very small subset of women who aren't healing well or have ongoing problems at 6 weeks postpartum, your midwife or doctor should continue providing ongoing care and/or appropriate medical referrals to experts until you're completely healed.

What about sex? Your doctor or midwife will check everything out at your postpartum checkup and let you know how it's progressing. If you need more healing time, you and your partner can explore some creative lovemaking that leaves your still-healing vagina out of the equation.

What if you had a really traumatic birth and have ongoing problems? A very small number of women experience urinary or fecal incontinence, sexual dysfunction, or pain long after birth. This is not normal. If you're having any incontinence at all, your provider should know about it. If you're having pain or trouble having sex, there's a lot of help available, including simple exercises and physical therapies. In fact, physical therapy to strengthen the pelvic floor and solve incontinence problems is a growing business. In France, they call this perineal reeducation, and it's part of routine postpartum care. It involves a series of exercise sessions and biofeedback techniques that help tone up the vagina and pelvic floor muscles to get everything back in shape for a healthy sex life, normal bladder and bowel control, and the ability to have healthy births in the future. We have these therapies here, too; they're just not as commonly available as in France.

What if you're healed and aren't having any pain or problems, but you just don't want to have sex yet? Don't worry about it. You've been through a lot. Your body, mind, and spirit have their own healing path on the road back to sexuality and you'll get there on your own time schedule. If you're worried about your lack of sexual desire, you might just need more time, but you might also benefit from some counseling with a therapist who specializes in maternal health.

Now that everything's different, will life ever be normal again?

Now that you've given birth and your heart has swelled to include your baby, will life ever be normal again? Will it be anything like it was Before Baby? In many ways, yes, it will be, but in many others, no freakin' way. Having a baby changes everything about how life works, how you approach day-to-day activities, and how you relate to the world outside your nursery, even though many elements of your life will remain the same. It's a matter of perspective. Welcome to your new normal.

Take relationships, for instance. You'll be with the same partner, but now he or she is a parent, too. You'll discover things about him or her that you didn't know or see before. You'll create new rituals and memories together and have entirely new things to talk about, plan for, and dream of. You'll have the same friends, but now you'll have to include your baby or make childcare arrangements before you hang out. If they're parents too, you'll finally get why they always wanted to talk about their kids. If they're not, you'll hope they understand why you can't stay up all night anymore. You'll make new friends, who are also new parents, and some of your old friends will drift away, unable to maneuver the changes your baby makes in your relationship. You'll still be a sister, daughter, and wife, but now you are also a mother, looking at the world through brand-new eyes. You'll still be a coworker, but now you'll be one of those with baby pictures on her desk.

How about that career of yours? For some of you, you'll still have your job but now you'll need childcare and while you're working, your baby will always be on your mind. You'll have to perform even when your toddler is teething and you've been awake all night. Or you may decide to leave the career you had and stay home while your baby is little. Or maybe your baby is providing the kick in the pants you needed to negotiate more flexible hours. Having a child creates all kinds of new necessities—which, as we know, is the mother of invention—and you may find yourself more motivated and inspired than ever before to create the conditions to do your best work.

What if most of your day is spent at home? You'll do the same things as always, but now you'll do them with a baby on your hip. You'll still have free time (aka nap time), but now you'll be more selective about how you spend it. You'll learn to do chores while holding a baby. You'll parcel out activities to coincide with your baby's best hours, and you'll relish the moment when your partner comes home and you finally get a break.

You'll still be you, with all your talents, quirks, worries, and gifts, but having a baby dials everything up to the next level. You're almost guaranteed to be more thoughtful, because there's so much more at stake; more stressed, because there's so much more to juggle, worry about, and ponder. You'll laugh more, and your sense of humor will expand because babies are downright funny. You'll see the world as your baby will, for all its beauty and danger, weirdness and wonder, and all its heretofore unimaginable possibilities. If you ever doubted it, you'll now know for certain that hope and love are more important than anything else.

Will life ever be normal again? No, it won't. But seriously, after you've had your baby, you won't want it to be. For better or worse, richer or poorer, mother or father, the new normal of life with your baby is so much better.

CHAPTER 15

Having a New Baby

Now that there's a baby, how does it all work? Sleeping, feeding, caretaking—how do you do anything now that baby is onboard? Let's find out.

A word about day three

The third day and night after you have your baby can be a bumpy one. You and your baby may hit the wall on day two, or you may have a longer honeymoon period and it doesn't happen until day four, but for most new mothers, day three is the rough one. That's the day when your milk comes in, the day you'll probably have to poop for the first time after birth, the day when you realize that life without real sleep is your new normal, and the day when your body is still achy and your mind is muddled and you thought you'd be feeling better than this. You've got hormones shifting from here to eternity, and your emotional stability is shot to hell.

Your baby isn't going to be feeling much better. This is the day when many of them figure out that this life-outside-the-womb thing is permanent. They come out of the fog a little, and while they find their parents charming, they're not too keen on the indignities of life. Day three is often when babies get pissed off and make sure their parents know it.

Day three is usually when your breasts take on a life of their own as they figure out how to produce enough milk to keep your baby alive. Most women's breasts are overachievers, and when the milk first comes in they will produce enough to feed all the children in the village. They'll be engorged, swollen, and achy. Your nipples may be bruised and cracked. The hormonal shifts and swelling that happen when your milk comes in can give you a low-grade fever and aches and pains. Use ice packs (bags of frozen peas are great) for 5 to 10 minutes before and after nursing and apply a heating pad for a few minutes before nursing to help your your milk flow. You can also take some ibuprofen or Tylenol. If your nipples are sore, use organic lanolin cream, burn-gel patches, or even a nipple shield to help them heal. Talk to a lactation nurse for specific tips.

The best way to deal with the engorgement of day three is to nurse your baby as often as possible, but don't be surprised if he's not nursing as much as he did on day one or two. Since he's now getting a volume of milk and not just a wee bit of colostrum, his tummy may stay fuller longer, and the two of you will need to adjust. If your breasts are unbearably full, go ahead and pump or hand-express just enough to get relief, but don't pump too much. Your breasts respond to the law of supply and demand. The more you nurse (or pump), the more milk you'll produce. If you pump too much, your breasts will interpret that as needing to make more.

Day three is also very often the day when you finally have a bowel movement, which means your sore perineum has to get back to the work of expelling waste from your body. If you've been keeping up with your fruit, veggie, and water consumption, you shouldn't be constipated. Hospitals hand out stool softeners like Pez for just this reason. Even if you are constipated, don't worry; you're unlikely to hurt yourself or break your stitches.

By day three, mothers who've had a vaginal birth are already home, and they don't have nurses around to help them. Mothers who've had a C-section are usually still in the hospital (or are going home on day three), but they're expected to participate in baby care. If day three seems like an unfairly rough transition to the realities of motherhood, I hope it helps you to know that day four is usually better and day five better still. How do you deal with your cranky baby; achy, exhausted body; sore bottom; and ridiculously productive breasts? As gently as possible.

Just know this is likely to be a tough day, that every mother goes through this, and that your baby's not having a great time either. Ask for extra help and support and tissues. If you find yourself crying and feeling vulnerable and a wee bit anxious, you're right on track and exactly where we expect you to be. Don't worry, mama—it's going to be OK.

What you can do the first week, second week, third week, sixth week

The first few weeks and months after having your baby offer real-time lessons in contrast—you're exhilarated and exhausted, joyous and anxious, aching and relieved. You've reached your goal, only to realize you've only just begun. After 9 months (or longer) of dreaming about the day when your baby is in your arms, you find yourself asking your-self *Now what?* So let's figure that out. What can you do in the first few weeks as a postpartum mom?

Week one—During the immediate days following birth (including that challenging day three, which we've discussed), your body has the multiple responsibilities of healing, making milk, and learning how to survive sleep deprivation. If it's your first baby, you won't have any idea what you're doing, yet you're expected to take responsibility for the most vulnerable person you've ever met. Your priorities during this first week of motherhood should be (1) supporting your body to heal and make milk and (2) learning the basics of baby care. That's it. You're not supposed to be taking care of anyone else, doing your housework, cook-ing dinner, exercising—nada. This first week should be spent this way: eat, drink, nurse, change the baby, sleep, repeat.

If this isn't your first baby, you'll obviously need to incorporate your other kid(s) into this routine, but you shouldn't be expected to take care of them yourself. This week of self-care and rest can be accom-plished only if you have support—your partner at home, a doula, your mother or sister or somebody else who is dedicated to taking care of you. What happens if you don't have that support? You'll be tempted to get up and around sooner than you should, and that's going to impact your ability to heal. If you don't have help, you still have to dedicate the first week to doing as little as possible. Same routine as for the new moms. Oh, and go ahead and toss in a daily shower, bath, or sponge bath, but then, seriously, that's all.

Week two—If you had a vaginal birth, you'll be feeling pretty close to back on your feet, or as good as you can feel on a few hours of interrupted sleep. Your vagina should have recovered from the worst of the swelling, and your lacerations should be healing well. If you had a C-section, your incision probably won't hurt much anymore and it will be knitting itself together well. Your vaginal bleeding will have dwindled to an annoying dribble, and your breasts will have learned they don't have to feed every baby in town, just yours. This is the week, however, when sleep deprivation piles up at the same time that most of your hands-on help disappears. Your baby will go through her first major growth spurt, and she'll want to nurse more frequently than usual. It's hard for your brain to figure out what's up—you're feeling better, and you're totally wiped out. You've got the hang of newborn care, and you're emotionally unprepared to handle it all alone. What's that cycle you should repeat? Eat, drink, nurse the baby, change a diaper, take a short walk, eat, drink, nurse, change, putter, sleep, and not much else. Don't worry too much about housework and laundry. Do the bare minimum you can get away with and still feel like you're civilized.

Note to dads and partners—yes, we know you're suffering from sleep deprivation and the stresses of new parenting, but your body isn't trying to heal and produce milk, so you do have to take care of everything that's not in mom's cycle. Housework? That's you. Laundry? You again. Cooking, shopping, schlepping your other kids to and fro? That's right—it's you. Don't worry: by week three, mom will be further along on the healing spectrum and will be able to do a wee bit more.

Week three—This is the week many women feel like they're either hitting their stride or hitting the skids. It all depends on how you deal with two things: sleep deprivation and the demands of taking care of a newborn. There's really no way to know in advance of becoming a parent how you'll cope with newborn-induced sleep loss. It's not like any other kind of sleep deprivation you've ever experienced. Not like the days when you'd go out dancing until all hours, then get up early for work. It's not like college, when you crammed all night for finals. It's not even like working night shift as a nurse, because at least then you could sleep for six or so hours during the day.

Sleep deprivation with a new baby is like this: You sleep with one eye open, because you're always on alert to make sure your baby is breathing. Then, on the off chance you go deep (REM sleep), you'll be woken up every hour and a half to two hours with someone screaming at you. The baby won't want much—a change, a meal, and a cuddle will usually do it—but there's no guarantee she'll go back to sleep. Therefore, neither will you. Babies don't know that nighttime means sleep and daytime means play, and while it's totally sweet that she wants to gaze at you and hear your voice at 3 A.M., it's also exhausting. And that meal she wants means you're breastfeeding for 20 minutes to an hour. This is the cycle you repeat now—sleep, wake, nurse, sleep, wake, nurse—all night long. When daytime hits, your baby will continue this cycle, but you'll be expected to do your daytime thing.

The demands of newborn care begin to add up during week three, too. You're back on task for doing at least some of the housework, cooking, and laundry, and it's no easy feat considering how often your baby nurses and needs to be changed and the fact that she's totally helpless without you. Add to that how little sleep you're getting. For some mothers, it's too much. Many moms are also realizing how much they miss their premotherhood life when they were able to come and go as they pleased, take a shower whenever they wanted, and spend their days with coworkers and adults who were interesting. They're used to accomplishing something by the end of their workday, and they're bewildered that after a day of mothering, there's not much to show for it.

Week three is when I recommend women do three things:

1. **Take stock.** Remember that what you accomplish by the end of your day is your child's survival and development as a human being. Don't take those things for granted. Your baby cannot survive without you, and her introduction to the world and her ability to learn how it works is all courtesy of you (and, yes, your partner). Pat yourself on the back, and don't worry if you can't get anything else done.

2. **Go find some friends.** In the village model of parenting, mothers have their sisters, aunties, and girlfriends nearby to share the load, keep them company, and give them a clue. If you don't have your own village already well established, go to the park, join a new moms' group at the hospital or a mother-baby yoga class, go out for lunch with a girlfriend (baby in tow, or watched over by others at home), attend story time at the library, or go wherever else mothers hang out in your community. When I was a brand-new mom with two babies under age 2, I placed an ad in the local children's bookstore that I was forming a playgroup and looking for other mothers. Four women responded, and two of them are still great friends today. We got together a few times a week to talk, drink coffee, and hang out. We created our own village, and thank god for that, because without these women, I'd have gone mad.

3. **Get some gentle exercise.** Nothing lifts a mood or battles fatigue better than exercise. You're not yet ready for a serious workout, but a walk in the neighborhood is perfect. Move your body, get some air, be outside, and reconnect with life outside the four walls of your nursery or living room.

If you find you're getting depressed, angry, anxious, or apathetic, those are all signs of postpartum depression. Check in with your midwife or doctor; ask your family and support people for help.

Six weeks—Your mood and energy level will depend greatly on your ability to survive without sleep and cope with the demands of newborn care. The good news is that by this time most babies have a clue about the difference between daytime and nighttime hours. Most are far more efficient about nighttime feedings, so you'll likely be getting a bit more sleep. You'll also have lost a chunk of pregnancy weight, and your body will almost be getting back to normal. You'll have your baby-care rhythm down, and you'll probably be feeling pretty confident.

For many women, the biggest hurdle they face now is their return to work. Personally, I think this is brutal and one of the worst things we do to American mothers. Since as of this writing we still don't offer paid maternity leave here in the United States, many women can't afford to stay home from work any longer, which means that even though their baby is still 100-percent dependent on them and they're still not getting enough sleep, they have to find childcare, leave their baby, go back to work, pump milk or wean to the bottle, and be professional. For some women, that's fine. They're ready to get back to work. For most, though, this is a huge challenge.

Six weeks is also when women return to their doctor or midwife for their final postpartum checkup. This is the biggie where they officially "graduate" from pregnancy and postpartumhood and get the green light to have sex. That's stressful for many women who aren't feeling entirely comfortable in their bodies yet, what with the weight they're still carrying, still feeling sore and vulnerable about sexual activity, their breasts that have their own thing going on, and of course, the fatigue, which is like a third member of their relationship. If you are one of those who aren't ready to have sex yet, it's important to realize you're normal. Your body's been through a lot, and you may need more time. Don't rush it, but do talk to your doctor about birth control, because you never know—you might be ready sooner than you expect.

Some women are ready to be sexual again. It allows them to reclaim their body as their own and to recognize themselves as a woman and a sexual being in addition to being a mother. It's a way to reconnect with their partner after weeks of attachment primarily to the baby. It's a way to allow their body pleasure after months of productivity. This is normal, too. My final word on this: birth control. Get some, unless you want back-to-back babies. That thing about not being able to get pregnant while breastfeeding? That's dangerous misinformation— you certainly can, and plenty of women do. In fact, I did.

Sleep, sleep deprivation, and how to keep from losing your mind

Unless you're among the minority of mothers who have nighttime help (baby nurse, doula, grandmother), you're in for a bit of a shock. Babies rule the night. They're totally clueless about circadian rhythms and not the least bit concerned about waking you up at all hours to make you do things for them. This goes on for months and months—sometimes even years.

Everyone will tell you: Sleep when the baby sleeps. That's excellent advice the first week or so but not so great after that, because few of us have the privilege of putting everything in life on hold while we take a nap.

We each react differently to interrupted and reduced sleep. Some can suck it up and function fairly well; others fall apart completely. They can't think, can't deal, and can't function at all. These parents have to create coping strategies to keep from losing their minds.

First, consider this: while it may seem like you're never getting to sleep, the reality is you're almost certainly getting some. Even if your baby is an every-two-hour feeder, that gorgeous hour and a half between feedings might drop you into the deepest sleep of your life. The body is amazing in its ability to grab what it needs, and once you get into a nighttime groove, you'll find the experience of having bizarre wake-sleep cycles less jolting.

If the fatigue is too extreme, then you and your partner need to make some changes—like alternating nights where one of you gets to sleep all night in a room away from the baby while the other handles night duties. If you're breastfeeding, this could involve your partner giving the baby a bottle of pumped milk or having dad bring baby in for a quick nighttime feeding, then scooping her back up and away while you go back to sleep.

Even when I'd been a nightshift nurse for quite some time, I found newborn sleep deprivation to be a special kind of awful. I didn't really mind nursing the baby in the middle of the night. In fact, I found it mighty cozy. It was the getting out of bed to get the crying baby that I just plain hated. So my husband and I would share the load. He'd get up and get the baby, do a diaper change, and tuck the baby in bed next to me. After she nursed, my husband would take the baby back to her bassinet. Neither one of us was gaining any extra sleep that way, but this system worked for us.

For some women, sleep deprivation leads to serious changes in mental health—aka postpartum depression and even psychosis. This is serious business and must be addressed by professionals—your doctor or midwife plus a psychologist, psychiatrist, or other mental health professional with experience dealing with postpartum mothers.

I had a touch of this with baby number one. I couldn't fall asleep for days after having my daughter. I was on high alert and pulsing with hormones, and my mind just would not let up. I'd doze a bit here and there but never really dropped off. One day, I was sitting in the rocker with my baby in my arms. She was asleep and I was exhausted. Suddenly, white horses were flying in her window. Whatever was left of my logical mind knew for certain this wasn't real, but all my other senses said, "My oh my, that sure is a lot of flying horses. I wonder what happens when they land." That was my only real break from reality, and shortly after the horses arrived, I was finally able to fall asleep.

Most parents gradually adapt to their life sans sleep. Week by week babies lengthen the hours between feedings. A few even sleep through the night by 6 weeks. Certainly none of my babies ever did that, but I've heard of babies that do. Eventually, they'll go to bed in the evening and wake up before dawn and you'll call that a good night's sleep.

Families find their own ways of dealing with the sleep thing. Some choose a family bed or cosleeping; although many pediatricians frown on this, billions of families throughout history and around the world have found it to be their best solution. Pediatricians' concerns stem from tragedies in which a baby is smothered when a parent rolls over on her or suffocates in heavy blankets. They're also concerned that babies will develop sleep disorders if they don't learn to fall asleep on their own. These are serious and valid concerns, yet parents who make the cosleeping choice say that babies are actually safer and sleep better when they sleep with their parents by their side. I think families have to work this out for themselves, and I encourage them to find the solution that matches their family's needs. If their pediatrician isn't happy with their arrangement, but the baby is thriving and the family is happy, well then, I'd say mom and dad know best.

We handled it like this: I learned early on that if the brand-new baby was in my bed, I wouldn't fall asleep. If she was in a Moses basket or bassinet next to my bed, I would. When she was too big for the bassinet, we moved her to a crib in the hall outside our door or in a bedroom nearby. By the time each of our kids was 6 months old, more or less, they were sleeping in their own room and waking us up only once a night. My husband and I took turns at crack o' dawn duty so each of us could catch up on a couple of hours' sleep. This is what worked for us, and over the years we learned that some kids needed more nighttime parenting than others. Some had trouble falling asleep. Some were big dreamers. One was a sleepwalker and another hated sleeping alone so she'd crawl into bed with a sibling or with us. Eventually they all worked it out, and nobody died from being tired.

I'm sure many pediatricians will disagree with me on this, but newborn sleep disruptions are temporary and maybe the best advice is to just do whatever it takes to get through the night. Somebody ought to write a love song about that.

How to do anything now that you have a newborn—including taking a shower, going to the store, and having an adult conversation

Babies have huge needs and never-ending demands. Many mothers want to be the number one person in their child's life, so they try to do it all even when there's help available. We have this whacked-out idea that what it takes to be a good mom is to sacrifice everything for your child. Here are my best pieces of parenting advice: Don't go over the top doing so much for your baby by yourself that you neglect your own needs. Don't make your partner an accessory or assistant—he or she is a coparent. Don't give 100 percent of yourself to your baby. Save some for yourself, some for your partner, and some for the rest of your life.

Parents usually come in sets of two (or if they don't, there are usually grandparents, aunts, uncles, and friends around to help), and both are important, capable, and perfectly suited to taking care of a baby. When mom tries to do it all and dad is treated like her little helper, this breeds resentment in both parents and wears mom out. It doesn't do the baby any good, either.

We all know women who complain about how little their partners do. They harp about having to do it all because he or she can't do anything well enough. They're pissed about being the primary parent and insist their partner won't do anything around the house without being nagged. They're angry when their partner does something differently than they would, or that they didn't specifically tell their partner to do. They're damned if they do and damned if they don't.

Whenever I encounter one of these women, I wonder how this situation developed. Why didn't she share the parenting load from day one and respect his contribution so they'd have a more equal partnership? What part did each of them play in reaching this point?

It's a weird cultural dynamic we have, but one that desperately needs to change. Unless both parents are enabled and empowered to be their child's caretaker from day one, mothers will take on too much and resent doing it all. Dads will check out because they feel like they're not good enough.

It's not just moms who put this dynamic into play. Society is all over it, too. It starts in the delivery room when dads are chided by nurses not to drop the baby or they're teased about a sloppy diaper change. Nobody does that with mom, because even if she has no baby experience, it's assumed she'll know how to hold her own child. It happens when they get home, when baby cries in dad's arms and mom insists he hand the baby over so she can soothe it. It continues when mom micromanages how dad provides basic care and criticizes him when he doesn't do things her way.

It happens when mom won't hand the baby over to dad long enough to take a shower or run to the store. Sure, the baby might cry, but dad can hone his comforting skills. It happens when dad's play style is different from mom's. Sure it's different, but children can learn and have fun with both parents. Later still, it happens when mom "takes care" of the children but dad "babysits" or "helps." All those subtle things lead too many women to thinking they don't have support, that they're the only one who can do anything. All of this tells dads they're not expected to take care of their own children.

But none of that is necessary. It's not true that dads aren't as capable of parenting as moms. They do things differently, for sure, but so what? (Moms don't all do it the same way, either.) Children are better off when they learn to adapt to more than one style and one parent. It's how they learn trust, adaptability, diversity, and strong but flexible gender roles.

So back to the original idea: How *can* you do anything now that you have a newborn—including taking a shower, going to the store, and having an adult conversation? You ask for help and accept it. You hand the baby to your partner and go take a shower. Take your time. Heck, shave your legs if you want to. Your baby will be fine. Go to the grocery store and leave your baby in your mother's care. Go ahead and dawdle over magazines. Make time to spend with your friends, your partner, and even all by yourself. You will always be your child's mother, but that doesn't mean you have to do it all. Your child deserves to have other adults in his life too, and he deserves to have a mother who is her own person.

The second baby— how to add another kid to your life

Among my biggest worries during my second pregnancy were these: I loved my first baby so much that I couldn't imagine I could love the next one as much. I worried my one-year-old would feel like I might if my husband brought home another wife. I imagined her thinking *Huh? Wasn't I good enough? You had to bring home someone else?*

Yeah, I know—kinda nutso. My sister screwed my head back on straight by reminding me that having another baby didn't take anything away from my firstborn daughter. Instead, I was giving her a gift—a sibling who would be a witness to her life, a playmate and first friend. Once I got over all my emotional concerns, I realized that my real worries were mostly strategic and practical—the how-to of feeding, bathing, raising, playing with, and affording an additional child. I checked out books from the library like *Your Second Child*,[1] which provided some excellent tips, and then I learned the same way most mothers do: by trial and error. I watched other mothers and absorbed tricks of the trade. Eventually, having two felt as natural as having one. Later, we added more kids, and again I felt a bit like you do in the first weeks at a new job. And then I adjusted. So will you.

CHAPTER 16

Feeding Your Baby

Breast? Bottle? A little of each? Pumping? Dumping? Nipple cream? Nursing pads? How are you going to feed that baby? That's what we'll talk about in this section.

Breast versus bottle—
battle lines and peace treaties

Everybody knows that breast is best. There's really no debate there. Nothing you can buy in a can will ever be better than the stuff you make with your very own breasts. Breast milk is superior in nutrition, antibodies, affordability—everything. Except when it's not. Then bottle feeding is better.

Now, before you go to war here about breast versus bottle (which, by the way, is the number one topic women comment on in my blogs), let's get real. Almost all women *can* breastfeed, even the ones with small breasts, inverted nipples, twins, triplets, mastitis—*almost* all women. We're built that way. If you're nourished and hydrated and nurse your baby often enough, you'll almost certainly make more than enough milk to feed your baby. Unless you can't, don't want to, or shouldn't.

Who are those women, the ones who can't breastfeed or don't want to? There are lots of us out there—that's right, I said "us." I breastfed my first three babies for a year or two each. I nursed my first while pregnant with my second. I nursed through mastitis, working the night shift, even when giving a bottle would have helped my husband bond with his babies. I was absolutely in the "breast is always best" camp until three months after I had baby number four.

From the day she was born, I hated nursing with my left breast. It irritated me and made me anxious. Right breast—no problem. I used both breasts, made enough milk, and didn't give my weird left breast aversion much thought, until my baby was three months old and I was diagnosed with breast cancer (in that left breast). I had three days to wean her before all kinds of nasty tests and treatments barreled down on me and, just like that, I switched teams. So much for my "breast is best" stance. It wasn't best for my baby or me anymore.

Over the many years I worked at the hospital, countless women confided in me that they felt like bad mothers because they didn't want to breastfeed. Some were rape survivors. Some had to return to work within a few weeks and didn't want to or wouldn't be able to pump. Some had had breast reduction surgery that had disrupted their milk glands. There were other reasons too, but it all boiled down to physical, emotional, or financial matters that meant breast was not best for them. Most felt pretty bad about it, like they weren't good mothers. If their reluctance to breastfeed was based on misinformation (my breasts are too small, or my mother couldn't breastfeed), I'd fuel them with education and encourage them to give it a try. If they were certain, though, I learned not to judge. That lesson in acceptance became crystal clear after I became a bottle feeder.

It's easy to judge other mothers and their parenting choices until you've walked a mile wearing her bra. If you've decided that breast is best for you, excellent. If you've decided formula is what you prefer, you've got my support. You've got your reasons, as I had mine, and we're both excellent mothers.

Let's call an end to this particular battle of the so-called mommy wars. Let's support all mothers in the choices they make, whether they align with ours or not. Let's support women to make the breastfeeding choice whenever possible, because we know that most of the time breast is absolutely a better nutritional choice than formula. Let's work together so women can get the lactation support they need. Let's create better maternity leave and work policies so women don't have to choose between breastfeeding and supporting their families. Let's knock off all the nonsense about picking on women who nurse in public. And then let's support the mothers who choose the bottle just as much. Seriously, whatever choice you make is perfectly OK.

How to get the help you need when breastfeeding is hard

You'd think it would come naturally, like any mammal can do it, right? Not so. Breastfeeding isn't always a piece of cake. Some babies are born exhausted, confused, and unable to latch. They can't get the hang of sucking, swallowing, and breathing in rhythm. Nipples come in funny shapes, too big or too small for a little mouth to latch onto without practice. They crack, chafe, blister, and bleed. Milk comes in too quickly or too slowly. Mothers are tired; babies are tired. Sometimes it's really hard.

Many women intend to breastfeed thinking it will be as simple and natural as taking off their shirt. Then they hit a wall, in the early days or weeks, or even months down the line. When someone recommends they "just give the baby a bottle," and baby figures out the bottle delivers milk more easily and faster than the breast, breastfeeding seems like a hassle. When nipples crack and it's too painful to nurse, it's easy to give up. When you have to go back to work and there's no time or place to pump in private or a really good pump is too expensive, well then, what's a mother to do? Call in a lactation support team!

Maybe the support you need is your mother or sister who prevailed against all breastfeeding odds. Maybe it's your postpartum nurse, who knows where the organic lanolin and cracked nipple supplies are stored. Maybe it's your midwife, who prescribes antibiotics when your milk ducts get plugged and infected, or a certified lactation consultant, who knows every trick in the book to bust through breastfeeding barriers. Maybe it's your human resources director, who can create provisions and work accommodations to support your efforts to pump. There are a lot of people out there who can help you make it work, as long as you ask for help.

For early struggles while you're in the hospital with your newborn, ask your nurses for help. They work with new mamas all day long. If their tips don't help, ask for a lactation nurse. They're the breastfeeding gurus who know what to do both when you're brand new at breastfeeding and when you've been at it a while. All major hospitals employ lactation consultants. You may also be able to get the help you need through online or video-chat support. Look for a local chapter of La Leche League. In some communities, home health nurses will come to your house and coach you through the rough patches.

Sometimes the only help you need comes in the form of personal support. Tell your family, friends, and partner that breastfeeding is extremely important to you. Ask them not to suggest bottle feeding. Tell them you're fully aware that formula exists and you know where to buy it. Tell them that when you're frustrated and struggling, the help you need is something to drink, a neck rub, a shoulder to cry on, encouragement, someone to buy nipple cream, a nap, a snack, some chocolate, a ride to the lactation clinic.

Most breastfeeding problems are solvable. Ask for help. Be resourceful, persistent, and patient. Check with your insurance provider to find out about coverage for breastfeeding supplies and services (that's a new perk of the Affordable Care Act) and stick with it.

Cracked, sore nipples? Engorgement? Tips for making your breasts feel better

Breastfeeding gives your nipples the workout of a lifetime. I don't care what kind of sex life you've had—unless you've had a baby before, your breasts have never had the amount of attention they'll get while breastfeeding a baby. There's nothing else like it. It's intense, and sometimes, ahem, it sucks. In fact, sometimes it's enough to make a grown woman call it quits on something she thought would be a pleasure.

Rumor has it that breastfeeding should never hurt, that under normal circumstances it should feel entirely natural. I disagree. Most women shouldn't have great trouble, but I think more women than not have at least a small period of adjustment as their breasts and nipples get used to their new duties. Cracked, chapped, and sore nipples are common for many women in the first days and weeks of nursing. If a woman can persevere through the first three weeks, she'll generally have breastfeeding nailed.

Many of the most common early nipple problems (cracking, bruising, bleeding) have to do with "latch"—the physical connection between mom's nipple and baby's mouth. If the nipple doesn't line up properly, or baby doesn't have enough in his mouth, or it rubs on the wrong part of his palate, or he sucks on the same part of the nipple over and over again, the nipple can suffer all kinds of abuse. When you reposition baby's mouth or the nipple and you improve his latch, the nipple is less irritated. Your postpartum nurse will help you with a few basic techniques like these:

- Get as much of your nipple into baby's mouth as possible—all the way up to the areola (the colored part that surrounds the nipple). Grasp your nipple with your fingers in a "C" or "U" shape to guide it into baby's mouth.

- Bring your baby to your breast rather than reaching forward to bring your breast to her.

- Switch positions with each feeding—cradle hold, cross hold, football hold, side lying, repeat. Alternate positions between feedings so different sections of the nipple get sucked on.

- Support your baby with a breastfeeding pillow or a couple of bed pillows with a blanket folded on top. You want baby's head, mouth, and spine to be aligned with your breast so he doesn't pull it down as he sucks to keep it in his mouth.

If these basics aren't enough, ask your nurse for advice on what else to do. She'll have a few ways to tweak your latch to perfection. She may also recommend you use organic medical-grade lanolin ointment on your breasts between feedings, to moisturize, soothe, and protect them from further chafing. I'm a huge fan of burn gel bandages to help heal cracked nipples quickly. You can pick them up in the drugstore and cut them down to fit your abrasion or crack. Remove them for feedings and replace them as soon as you're done. More natural techniques include placing cabbage leaves in your bra, applying wet tea bags, and allowing breast milk to dry on the nipple. If all else fails or your nipples are inverted or oddly shaped, give nipple shields a try. These plastic flexible nipple-shaped discs fit over the nipple during nursing and between feedings. When baby latches on, it draws your nipple into the shield and lets baby breastfeed without irritating your nipple. You may not need the shields for long. Once your baby gets the basics of nursing down, you'll likely be able to wean him from the shield.

If your nipples are red, itchy, or have a rash, you may have a yeast infection or other type of infection. See your doctor and get a prescription to treat your breasts and your baby's mouth. If you have yeast, your baby has thrush (caused by the same yeast organism), and unless you're both treated, you'll just pass it back and forth. Make sure your bra is dry and clean and you change your breast shields frequently.

Engorgement means breasts are so full of milk and extra circulation that they become huge, hard, tight, and painful. This is super common when milk first comes in, on about postpartum day three. Sometimes there's so much inflammation, women even run a low-grade fever. The best way to deal with it is to encourage your baby to nurse as often as possible. Sometimes, however, baby is suddenly confronted with more milk volume than he's been getting with colostrum. He gets full quickly and nurses less often than mom needs to drain her breasts. In that case, you may need to hand express or pump just enough milk to relieve the pressure, but not so much that your breasts think you need to make more milk. Take ibuprofen and use ice packs and warm compresses or a hot shower to relieve discomfort, and don't hesitate to wake your baby up for feedings. All that milk is for him, after all.

If these DIY tips don't fix you and your girls up, get professional help. Ask your midwife or doctor to hook you up with a lactation consultant.

Pumping, dumping, storing, and freezing your breast milk

Maybe you're making more milk than your baby needs or you want to store some for date night. Maybe you're pumping at work so your nanny can feed your baby. Maybe you're ready for a party night (a glass of wine!) but don't want your baby to partake. Maybe you make enough milk to feed a small village and you want to donate to the milk bank. Whatever the reason, pumping breast milk is in your future.

It's entirely possible to express all the milk you want just by using your own hands. It's not that hard to learn; any mom can do it. Mothers throughout history all over the world have hand expressed and done just fine. When the portable breast pump was invented sometime in the mid-nineteenth century, however, and later, when modern refrigeration was invented, women realized that a good breast pump made the job easier, faster, and more comfortable and practical. The ability to store breast milk meant for the first time in history breastfeeding mothers had the ways, means, and freedom to spend a few hours away from their baby without needing a wet nurse.

The first breast pump models were big and clunky and found only in hospitals. For the last forty years or so, they've been available for rent or purchase and have become part of many nursing mothers' arsenal. Nowadays they're sleek, lightweight, crazy-efficient, travel well in a tote bag, and empty a breast at warp speed (OK, actually in about 10 minutes, but still, that's pretty good). Even better, the Affordable Care Act mandates that insurance providers have to cover breast pumps and breastfeeding supplies for all nursing mothers.

Once you've pumped your milk, you'll need to store it. You can purchase plastic breast milk bags and pouches or use zip-locking bags. Some women freeze their milk in ice cube trays. Others use glass or plastic bottles or other containers. If you're transporting milk home from work, you'll need a small cooler and a couple of portable ice packs. If you're going to use your pumped milk within a few days, store it in the refrigerator. If you're storing it for later use, freeze it.

Here are La Leche League's guidelines for breast milk storage:

All milk should be dated before storing. Storing milk in 2- to 4-ounce amounts may reduce waste. Refrigerated milk has more anti-infective properties than frozen milk. Cool down fresh milk in the refrigerator before adding it to previously frozen milk.

Preferably, human milk should be refrigerated or chilled right after it is expressed. Acceptable guidelines for storing human milk are as follows. Store milk:

- At room temperature (66–78°F, 19–26°C) for 4 hours (ideal), up to 6 hours (acceptable) (some sources say 8 hours)

- In a refrigerator (< 39°F, < 4°C) for 72 hours (ideal), up to 8 days (acceptable if collected in a very clean, careful way)

- In a freezer (–0.4 to –4°F, –18 to –20°C) for 6 months (ideal) up to 12 months (acceptable)

For storing human milk, follow these tips:

- Use glass or hard-sided plastic containers with well-fitting tops, not made with the controversial chemical bisphenol A (BPA)— wash in hot, soapy, water, rinse well, and allow to air-dry before use.

- Use freezer milk bags designed for storing human milk.

- Disposable bottle liners or plastic bags are not recommended. With these, the risk of contamination is greater. These bags are less durable and tend to leak, and some types of plastic may destroy nutrients in milk.

- Do not fill containers to the top—leave an inch of space to allow the milk to expand as it freezes.

- Put only 2 to 4 ounces (60 to 120 ml) of milk in the container (the amount your baby is likely to eat in a single feeding) to avoid waste.

- Mark the date on the storage container. Include your baby's name on the label if your baby is in a daycare setting.

What about alcohol and breastfeeding? We've been sending mixed messages on this for generations. Women used to be advised to drink beer to enrich their milk or wine to relax them while breastfeeding. More recently, women were told not to drink any alcohol, lest they get their baby drunk. Women who wanted to go out and have a couple of drinks would end their night by pumping and dumping their breast milk. Nowadays, we seem to have settled on more moderate guidelines for women who drink alcohol.

La Leche League's *The Womanly Art of Breastfeeding* (page 328) has this recommendation:

> *The effects of alcohol on the breastfeeding baby are directly related to the amount the mother ingests. When the breastfeeding mother drinks occasionally or limits her consumption to one drink or less per day, the amount of alcohol her baby receives has not been proven to be harmful.*[1]

And La Leche League's *The Breastfeeding Answer Book* (pages 597–598) says:

> *Alcohol passes freely into mother's milk and has been found to peak about 30 to 60 minutes after consumption, 60 to 90 minutes when taken with food. Alcohol also freely passes out of a mother's milk and her system. It takes a 120-pound woman about two to three hours to eliminate from her body the alcohol in one serving of beer or wine . . . the more alcohol that is consumed, the longer it takes for it to be eliminated. It takes up to 13 hours for a 120-pound woman to eliminate the alcohol from one high-alcohol drink. The effects of alcohol on the breastfeeding baby are directly related to the amount the mother consumes.*[2]

The American Academy of Pediatrics Committee on Drugs considers alcohol compatible with breastfeeding. Moderate amounts don't seem to be a problem at all. They warn women not to overdo it, because large amounts of alcohol can make babies sleepy and lethargic—and if consumption of breast milk with alcohol content is heavy and frequent, it can even make them overweight.

So, do you need to pump and dump? As long as you're drinking moderately and responsibly, probably not.

What if you want to donate milk to a breast milk bank? Check out the National Milk Bank at www.nationalmilkbank.org for qualifications and guidelines.

Bottle feeding, judgment free

Hey, honey—you have your reasons why bottle feeding is your thing, and I respect them. The only plug I'll make here for breastfeeding is this: If your reason for bottle feeding is based on fear, lack of information, or insecurity, I encourage you to ask for a little help and give it a try. Many women change their mind once they get into it. If you know, however, that you're not into breastfeeding, or you tried and it didn't work out, or you're going back to work and can't pump, or your health, lifestyle, or situation means breastfeeding isn't doable—OK by me. I've been there, and you totally have my support.

This section is all about how to make peace with the decision to bottle feed and how to keep haters off your back.

We're fortunate to live in a country where formula is high quality and easy to purchase and prepare and provides excellent nutrition for babies. We have clean water, a wide variety of bottles and nipples, and tons of formula options. You don't have to worry that your baby is getting shortchanged because she's getting a bottle instead of the breast. She'll be fine. She'll still get all the nutrition she needs, plus tons of holding, loving, and cuddling while you're feeding her. In fact, one of the bonuses of bottle feeding is that your partner can get in on all that snuggly feeding action, too.

It's the sad truth that some women are insecure about their own mothering skills or they think that good mothers fit in a one-size-only mold. They're proud of their choices and feel a bit superior about them. They build themselves up by spreading the gospel of their personal choices (breast versus bottle, natural versus epidural, and so on), and too often they come off as self-righteous, judgmental, opinionated, and pushy. These are the women who have no qualms about telling bottle-feeding mothers at the park, "Breast is best." They're the ones commenting loud and strong on breast-versus-bottle blogs, and usually in less than supportive terms. They think that sniping (with sweet tones and bless-your-hearts) at mothers who make different choices is somehow acceptable. Some even think they're being helpful, as if that poor bottle-feeding mother didn't realize what those things on her chest were there for. "If you want the best for your baby, you'd breastfeed." They're actually being quite narrow-minded. They're not thinking about why some women make different choices.

It's not your job to enlighten other women about why you bottle feed. But unless you have the patience of Mother Teresa and you don't mind explaining your decision to women, you may want to think up a couple of snappy comeback lines. Aim for short, sweet, and sassy. I'm afraid that when I bottle fed my youngest baby, I leaned toward snarky, bitchy, and hostile. I couldn't help it. I was sick, frustrated, and tired of women who didn't know my story dumping on me. I'm pretty sure you can do better. Here are a few you can use:

- I'm pro-choice, and I choose the bottle.

- Breast is best for you, but it isn't best for me.

- Don't I want the best for my baby? Of course I do. Don't you want to keep your snide remarks to yourself?

- Honor diversity, sister.

- Breast is best? You don't say. Maybe you'd like to spend the next hour with me while I explain my personal decision to you. No? Oh, well then, carry on.

My point is, you don't owe anyone an explanation, but it might help shut a few judge-y folks down (and make them think) if you have an answer that shows you know what you're doing and you're doing just fine thankyouverymuch. How about this one: No guilt, no judgment, no reason to argue about this, ladies. Some mothers choose breast, some choose bottle, and it's time we all supported each other.

How long should you breastfeed?

I like the American Academy of Pediatrics answer to the "How long should I breastfeed?" question:

> The AAP recommends that babies be exclusively breastfed for about the first 6 months of life. This means your baby needs no additional foods (except vitamin D) or fluids unless medically

indicated. Babies should continue to breastfeed for a year and for as long as is mutually desired by the mother and baby. Breastfeeding should be supported by your physician for as long as it is the right choice for you and your baby.[3]

This, of course, is the ideal—at least 6 months of breast milk only, followed by at least another 6 months of breastfeeding along with solid foods, followed by however long mom and baby are still into it. As long as mom and baby are happy, there really is no end date on how long they should breastfeed. One year, two years, longer—that's cool. Do what feels right to you, though be aware that in our culture many people are uncomfortable about mothers who nurse much past the second birthday. In other countries, breastfeeding toddlers and preschoolers is no big deal—nothing extreme or competitive about it. Mothers are just feeding their little ones in a cozy, lovely way.

What if you only want to breastfeed short term? Excellent! Colostrum (the first milk produced by the breasts) is chock-full of antibodies your baby needs to build up immunities to disease. Even if you nurse for only a few days, your baby will benefit; if you can go longer, even better. Go as long as you can and get as much help as you need to make that work. Quit when you have to or want to, and feel proud of however long it lasted.

How to work and breastfeed

Returning to work and continuing to breastfeed is 100-percent possible, as long as you have a few supplies, the support of your employer, and a place to pump. As soon as your pregnancy is official at your workplace, start the conversation with your human resources manager or boss about how you'll be breastfeeding at home and pumping at work. If you're lucky, your company will already have well-established policies in place and you won't have to be a breast pump pioneer. If you're the first, here's what you need to know:

Effective March 23, 2010, as mandated by the Patient Protection and Affordable Care Act of 2010, employers must provide break time and a place for hourly paid workers to express breast milk at work. The law states that employers must provide both a "reasonable" amount of time and a private space other than a bathroom. They are required to provide this until the employee's baby turns one year old.[4]

The "Break Time for Nursing Mothers" section of the law does not require pumping breaks to be paid. However, if your employer already offers paid breaks and you use those breaks to pump your milk, your time should be paid in the usual way. If you need extra time beyond what is usually allowed for these paid breaks, then the additional time does not need to be paid, and your employer may ask you to "punch out" for the additional time.

Employers with fewer than fifty employees are not required to comply with this law if it would impose an undue hardship (determined by looking at the difficulty or expense of compliance for a specific employer in comparison to the size, financial resources, nature, and structure of the employer's business).

What do you need to make it work?

A good breast pump (which should be covered by your insurance), collection supplies, a cooler, and ice packs. (See "Pumping, dumping, storing, and freezing your breast milk," page 212.)

How often should you pump?

As often as your baby eats. In the first few months, you'll need to pump about every 2 or 3 hours during your workday. As your baby gets older, that schedule may change, and it's important that you accommodate it as closely as possible to sync up with your baby's feeding schedule. If you don't nurse often enough, your milk supply will go down and you won't have enough to feed your baby. After your baby reaches 6 months, you can probably pump less often, since she'll be starting to eat solid foods.

Help your employer figure out how to accommodate for breaks and space to pump. Here our some solutions suggested by the U.S. Breast-feeding Committee:

Space solutions:

- Unused areas like a storage closet, empty office, or meeting room
- Manager's office
- Area that can be partitioned or blocked by a curtain
- Company or personal vehicle with window coverings
- Pop-up tents or temporary walls
- Working from home (if possible)

Break time solutions:

- Pumping during existing authorized breaks
- Coming in early or staying late to make up for lost time
- "Floating" staff to cover during pumping and other breaks (lunch, bathroom, etc.)
- Bringing a laptop or phone to the pumping space to continue working while pumping (if this works for you)
- Returning to work part-time (if possible)

I also like the committee's suggestions for how to talk to employers about accommodating breastfeeding. The chart outlines some of the most common objections moms hear when talking to their employer; these may help you consider and prepare for any concerns your employer may have. Ultimately, the answer to the most stubborn objections is, "Accommodating me is required by law."[5]

IF YOUR EMPLOYER SAYS . . .	TRY RESPONDING WITH . . .
"The bathroom is the only space available."	"Breast milk is food for my baby, so it shouldn't be expressed in a bathroom. I looked into some solutions that other companies have used that I think will work here too." [If needed: "Finding a space that isn't a bathroom is required by law."]
"How am I supposed to cover your position while you are on break?"	"I thought through a schedule and how we could handle it. It's actually pretty similar to how we handle other staff breaks—can I tell you what I have in mind?"
"This will be bad for business."	"Actually, a lot of companies say that it's *good* for business. Breastfeeding will help keep me and my baby healthy so I can do my best work."
"Why can't you just pump when you get home?"	"If I don't pump as often as my baby eats, my supply will go down, and I won't make enough to feed her. It's really important to me, and it's only temporary."
"My daughter/niece/friend drank formula and she's the smartest/ fastest/healthiest kid in her class."	"Lots of kids do! But this is really important to me and is recommended by the American Academy of Pediatrics. I can't do it without your support."
"I can't make any promises if it gets busy."	"I'm more than willing to be flexible, and I know we can make this work for both of us."

What if your boss and coworkers resent your "pump time"?

So what? Be a badass mama and do it anyway. You have a legal right to breastfeed your baby, and if that right isn't exercised, it's going to be weak for all mothers. Try to pump at times when your break is least disruptive, and remain as flexible as possible. Remember this: you may be the only nursing mama there today, but others will come along behind you. Consider yourself one of the pioneers who is improving workplace standards for all women.

Conclusion

Labor is over and you've had your baby, but really, it's only the beginning. Now is when you'll all grow into the new lives your pregnancy created—those of a mother, a father or partner, and a brand-new baby—your family. This is when you'll discover parts of yourself and your partner that you never knew existed. This is the new you, the better you, the one you always knew you would be.

Being a parent is guaranteed to be more fun, much harder, and way more rewarding than you every thought it would be. The fun will come in unexpected bursts, in messy, dusty, sticky play and glimpses of your baby as he grows into himself. It'll be silly, funny, and heartbreakingly beautiful. It will be as joyous as falling in love, except that there will be no holding back. You will love your child unconditionally, even when he drives you nuts. The hard part will be the fatigue, the anxiety, and the great unknown that is part of the fabric of parenting. Rest assured, though, that it's all doable. You'll have more resources and help than you know, as long as you have the good sense to reach out and ask for it.

And the reward? Oh, the reward. You know that feeling you get when you work really hard at a brand-new project and it totally turns out great? You know those work days that are so much longer and more complicated than you anticipated? The ones that were so interesting and challenging that the payback is in the work itself? Yeah, that's parenting. You're in for a good time, my friend.

Pregnancy and parenting for women with history: getting real about custody, child welfare, drug addiction, domestic violence, homelessness

There is no such thing as a perfect mother. Nobody has ever made it through life without screwing up in some minor or major way. We're human, and our personal histories accompany us into motherhood—even the incidents we're not entirely proud of.

Maybe we partied too hard or grew up surrounded by violence or angry parents. Maybe we got involved with the wrong guy or hung out with wild friends and did stuff we wish we hadn't. Maybe we were just normal women and nothing we ever did was a problem before we became pregnant. That's when everything changes. Suddenly, being a normal, wild, messed-up, or hard-partying woman isn't OK anymore. Suddenly, we're mothers in a society that has a limited standard for what constitutes good motherhood.

Just because some women don't stand under that very small umbrella that covers our society's definition of "good motherhood" doesn't mean they're not good mothers. Virtually all women love their children fiercely and want what's best for them. However, for some, circumstances have left them vulnerable. In the United States, few mothers are guaranteed all the financial, emotional, employment, and childcare support they need to be the best mothers possible, and some vulnerable mothers get very little support at all. There are services out there to help with addiction, unemployment, homelessness, and violence, but in such limited supply that many women living in desperate, disadvantaged circumstances can't access them.

What we need is a bigger umbrella that covers all mothers—even those who are less than perfect—one that recognizes we all need support, not judgment. If we do better at taking care of all mothers, then mothers can do better at taking care of their children.

What should you do if you're at risk and need help to be a good mother?

1. Whatever is making you vulnerable—fix it as best you can.

2. Ask for help—legal, emotional, financial, residential, educational. Getting help starts with reaching out.

3. Access parenting support classes.

4. If you're in danger, find safety—a shelter or sanctuary.

5. Build your community of supportive, solid people who can help you raise your children well.

6. Tell your story. The more women share their experiences, the bigger the umbrella that covers us all.

Finally, don't judge other mothers. None of us is perfect. We're all just doing the best we can. Some of us just have more to work with or work on than others.

When a Baby Dies

It's rare, but it happens, and it's devastating. It feels like there's something wrong with the natural order of the universe when the hope of a gorgeous baby is destroyed by death. Few parents recover from this easily, if they ever fully recover at all. All of them are left with an unanswerable question: Why?

Before we dig into the emotional, spiritual, and intellectual challenge of why babies die and what happens next, let's do the numbers:

According the Department of Health and Human Services, in 2009 (the most recent data at this writing) 17,298 infants died in the United States before reaching 28 days of age, representing a neonatal mortality rate of 4.19 deaths per 1,000 live births.[1] Neonatal mortality is generally related to short gestation (prematurity) and low birth weight, congenital malformations, and conditions originating in the perinatal period, such as maternal complications related to pregnancy or complications experienced by the newborn resulting from birth. And 9,233 infants died between the ages of 28 days and 1 year, representing a postneonatal mortality rate of 2.24 deaths per 1,000 live births.[2] These deaths are generally related to Sudden Infant Death Syndrome (SIDS), congenital malformations, and unintentional injuries.

According to the National Stillbirth Society, stillbirth is defined as the intrauterine death and subsequent delivery of a developing infant that occurs beyond 20 completed weeks of gestation. Stillbirth occurs in about 1 in 160 pregnancies. The majority of stillbirths happen before labor, whereas a small percentage occurs during labor and delivery.[3]

In about one-third of cases, the cause for stillbirth can't be determined, but the majority of deaths are related to placental problems, intrauterine growth restriction, infections, and birth defects. Very, very rarely it's caused by umbilical cord accidents, trauma, maternal diabetes, high blood pressure, and postdate pregnancy (a pregnancy that lasts longer than 42 weeks).

It's hard to know what to write about the devastating experience of losing a baby. In some ways it's like any death, and the normal patterns of grief will follow. But it's unlike any other death because it occurs at the beginning of life, when by rights the child and parents should have decades of life together in front of them. How does one grieve a baby whose life was cut so short that it barely had time to live? In the case of stillbirth, parents have to say goodbye before they ever say hello. It's unimaginably sad.

Parents are usually able to hold their stillborn baby for as long as they want. They should never be rushed to release the baby to the morgue. Whether it takes an hour or several days, most hospitals recognize that this is the only time these parents and this baby will have together, and nobody should shortchange them that time. Eventually the baby will be weighed, measured, bathed, and dressed, and footprints will be taken. The parents will be offered a lock of hair, the baby's first T-shirt and blanket, and other mementos. They'll be given information about funeral arrangements and autopsies and support groups and counselors. Family members will come and go, absorbing their own grief and attending to the family. They'll offer food, condolences, and advice. They'll offer to help, to cook, and to care for other children. It won't help the parents much, but it's what we do in times of loss and grief. The parents will be so sad, though, that they may not be able to accept what is offered. Eventually the mother will be discharged from the hospital and the baby will go to the morgue until the mortuary collects its body.

I've heard people say all kinds of things to parents during the early gruesome hours and days after their baby's death:

- It was God's plan.

- He's in a better place.

- She's with the angels now.

- At least you don't have to raise a deformed baby.

- Can you think of anything you did that caused this?

- At least you know you can get pregnant.

- You can have another baby right away.

People say these things because they don't know any other way to behave. They're thoughtless and heartless, but in a warped way, they usually come from a place of compassion. While almost anything said to the grieving family can be taken the wrong way, maybe the best thing to say is this: "I love you. I'm so sad. I'll be here with you in any way you need me." Then, be there. Be there for a long, long time, because this is a loss that will hurt for months, years, forever. Keep showing up. Keep being there.

One time, I was taking care of a mother who had just delivered her stillborn daughter. Her baby had been perfectly fine until 39 weeks, when suddenly she stopped moving. An ultrasound confirmed the worst possible news. The baby was dead. The mother was induced and delivered her baby vaginally. She held her in her arms for hours, staring at her thick red hair, stroking her eyebrows, and caressing her tiny, perfect hands. The father was unable to deal with his grief, shock, and pure rage; he left the room about an hour after the birth. This is not unusual. A father's primal job is to protect his family and fix problems, and for some men facing this kind of tragedy, their inability to do this job is just too much to deal with. Many men need time to gather themselves before they can be there for anyone else. This is normal.

The mother had been silent and tearless since her daughter's birth. Her parents were with her, but except for offering a few words of kindness, nobody seemed able to do much more than sit still. I'd ordered some food to be delivered to this mother's room, and when it arrived— delivered by the cook who had prepared it (a middle-aged man who'd been in the hospital kitchen for twenty years)—the tray was decorated with tiny white roses. News travels fast in hospitals, and he'd heard there'd been a stillbirth. He went to the gift shop, purchased the roses with his own money, and insisted on carrying the tray himself. Placing it on her bedside table, the cook said this: "Ma'am, there is nothing I can do that will relieve your pain, nothing I can do to make this easier for you to bear. These flowers will do nothing to make this better, but I brought them because I want you to know that people you will never know care deeply about you. I care, and in some little way, I hope that will ease your burden." That was the moment this mother finally started to cry. She hadn't been able to before this, but it was this man's pure kindness that broke the dam. She reached for his hand. He asked for permission to sit with her, and when she gave it, he simply sat in a chair beside her while she cried, holding her hand the whole time. He never said anything else to her. He just let her grieve and did what he could to absorb it. It was the single most graceful thing I've ever witnessed. A stranger, a devastated mother, a tray of food, some flowers, a few honest words, and a hand held as long as she wanted.

Notes and Resources

Chapter 1: When You First Get Pregnant

1. American Pregnancy Association, "Bleeding During Pregnancy," www.americanpregnancy.org/pregnancycomplications/ bleedingduringpreg.html.

2. "Length of Pregnancy by Weeks," SpaceFM.com, http://spacefem.com/pregnant/charts/duedate3.php.

3. "Definition of Term Pregnancy," The American Congress of Obstetricians and Gynecologists, The Society for Maternal-Fetal Medicine, Committee Opinion Number 579, November 2013.

Chapter 2: Choosing Your Care

1. American College of Nurse-Midwives, "Proportion of Midwife-Attended Births Reaches All-Time High in United States," www.midwife.org/JMWH-Midwife-Attended-Births.

2. S. Maher, A. Crawford-Carr, and K. Neidigh, "The Role of the Interpreter/Doula in the Maternity Setting," *Nursing for Women's Health* 16(6) (2012 Dec): 472–81.

3. H. A. Brouwers, W. Bruinse, J. Dijs-Elsinga, E. de Miranda, A. Ravelli, and P. Tamminga (eds.), *Netherlands Perinatal Registry: Perinatal Care in the Netherlands 2010* (Utrecht: Netherlands Perinatal Registry, 2013).

4. Unicef India Statistics, www.unicef.org/infobycountry/india_statistics.html.

5. Childbirth Connection, "Choosing a Place of Birth," www.childbirthconnection.org/article.asp?ck=10145.

6. O. Olsen and J. A. Clausen, "Planned Hospital Birth versus Planned Home Birth," *Cochrane Database System 9* (Rev. 2012, Sept. 12): CD000352.

7. Rebecca Dekker, "New Evidence Confirms Birth Centers Provide Top-Notch Care," American Association of Birth Centers (January 31, 2013).

8. Ibid.

Chapter 3: Your Pregnant Body

1. Centers for Disease Control, "Fact Sheet: Bacterial Vaginosis," www.cdc.gov/std/bv/stdfact-bacterial-vaginosis.htm

Chapter 4: Prenatal Tests

1. Eugenius S. B. C. Ang, Jr., Vicko Gluncic, Alvaro Duque, Mark E. Schafer, and Pasko Rakic, "Prenatal Exposure to Ultrasound Waves Impacts Neuronal Migration in Mice," Proceedings of the National Academ of Sciences of the United States of America www.pnas.org/content/103/34/12903.abstract?maxtoshow.

2. International Programme on Chemical Safety, "Environmental Health Criteria 22: Ultrasound, www.inchem.org/documents/ehc/ehc/ehc22.htm.

3. Guoyang Luo, and Errol R. Norwitz, "Revisiting Amniocentesis for Fetal Lung Maturity After 36 Weeks' Gestation," *Reviews in Obstetrics & Gynecology* 1(2) (2008 Spring): 61–68, www.ncbi.nlm.nih.gov/pmc/articles/PMC2505159.

Chapter 6: How to Deal with Late Pregnancy Curve Balls

1. March of Dimes, "Pregnancy Complications: Polyhydramnios," www.marchofdimes.com/pregnancy/polyhydramnios.aspx.

2. American Pregnancy Association, "Group B Strep Infection: GBS," http://americanpregnancy.org/pregnancycomplications/groupbstrepinfection.html.

3. Centers for Disease Control, "Group B Strep (GBS)," www.cdc.gov/groupbstrep/about/newborns-pregnant.html.

Chapter 7: When the End Is in Sight

1. Recent declines in induction of labor by gestational age. Osterman MJ, Martin JA. www.ncbi.nlm.nih.gov/pubmed?term=24941926.

2. D. Garry, R. Figueroa, J. Guillaume, and V. Cucco, "Use of Castor Oil in Pregnancies at Term," *Alternative Therapies in Health and Medicine* 6(1) (2000, Jan.): 77–9, www.ncbi.nlm.nih.gov/pubmed/10631825.

3. S. Azhari, S. Pirdadeh, M. Lotfalizadeh, and M. T. Shakeri, "Evaluation of the Effect of Castor Oil on Initiating Labor in Term Pregnancy," *Saudi Medical Journal* 27(7) (2006, Jul.): 1011–4, http://www.ncbi.nlm.nih.gov/pubmed/16830021.

4. J. Kavanagh, A. J. Kelly, and J. Thomas, "Breast Stimulation for Cervical Ripening and Induction of Labour," *Cochrane Database System Rev.* (3) (2005, Jul. 20): CD003392, www.ncbi.nlm.nih.gov/pubmed/16034897.

Chapter 10: Labor Pains

1. A. Pennell, V. Salo-Coombs, A. Herring, F. Spielman, and K. Fecho. "Anesthesia and analgesia-related preferences and outcomes of women who have birth plans," Journal of Midwifery & Women's Health. 2011 Jul-Aug;56(4):376–81.

2. National NHS Patient Survey Programme Survey of Women's Experiences of Maternity Services 2010 Full National Results Tables, The Care Quality Commission, www.cqc.org.uk/sites/default/files/documents/20101201_mat10_briefing_final_for_publication_201101072550.pdf.

Chapter 11: Other Labor and Delivery Issues

1. Steven L. Bloom, Brian M. Casey, Joseph I. Schaffer, Donald D. McIntire, Kenneth J. Leveno, "A Randomized Trial of Coached versus Uncoached Maternal Pushing during the Second Stage of Labor," *American Journal of Obstetrics and Gynecology* (2005 June), www.ajog.org/article/S0002-9378(05)00870-7/abstract-article-footnote-1Top of Form.

2. J. I. Schaffer, S. L. Bloom, B. M. Casey, D. D. McIntire, M. A. Nihira, and K. J. Leveno, "A Randomized Trial of the Effects of Coached vs Uncoached Maternal Pushing during the Second Stage of Labor on Postpartum Pelvic Floor Structure and Function," *American Journal of Obstetrics and Gynecology* 192(5) (2005 May): 1692–6, www.ncbi.nlm.nih.gov/pubmed/15902179.

3. V. L. Handa, T. A. Harris, and D. R. Ostergard, "Protecting the Pelvic Floor: Obstetric Management to Prevent Incontinence and Pelvic Organ Prolapse," *Obstet Gynecol* 88(3) (1996 Sept.): 470–8, www.ncbi.nlm.nih.gov/pubmed/8752261.

4. Placenta abruptio: Premature separation of placenta; Ablatio placentae; Abruptio placentae; Placental abruption, *A.D.A.M. Medical Encyclopedia*, www.ncbi.nlm.nih.gov/pubmedhealth/PMH0001903.

Chapter 12: C-Sections, VBACs, and More

1. "Ob Gyns Issue Less Restrictive VBAC Guidelines," American College of Obstetricians and Gynecologists (2010, July 21), www.acog.org/About_ACOG/News_Room/News_Releases/2010/Ob_Gyns_Issue_Less_Restrictive_VBAC_Guidelines?IsMobileSet=false.

2. Pitolese, R. (2002). "The Webster Technique: A chiropractic technique with obstetric implications." *Journal of Manipulative and Physiological Therapeutics*, Volumn 25, Issue 6, pages 1–9.

3. Ewies, A., and Olah, K. (2002). "Moxibustion in breech version—a descriptive review." *Acupuncture in Medicine*, 26–29.

Chapter 13: Once the Baby Is Born

1. Stanford School of Medicine, "Guidelines for Vitamin K Prophylaxis," http://newborns.stanford.edu/VitaminK.html.

Chapter 15: Having a New Baby

1. Joan Solomon Weiss, *Your Second Child* (New York: Summit Books, 1981).

Chapter 16: Feeding Your Baby

1. Wiessinger, D., and West, D. (2010). *The Womanly Art of Breastfeeding* (8th ed., p. 328). New York: Ballantine Books.

2. Mohrbacher, N., and Stock, J. (2003). *The Breastfeeding Answer Book* (3rd rev. ed., pp. 597–598). Schaumburg, Ill.: La Leche League International.

3. American Academy of Pediatrics, "Breastfeeding Initiatives FAQs," www2.aap.org/breastfeeding/faqsBreastfeeding.html

4. United States Breastfeeding Committee, "How Often Can You Pump during the Workday?" www.usbreastfeeding.org/Employment/WorkplaceSupport/WorkplaceSupportin FederalLaw/HowOftenCanPump/tabid/366/Default.aspx.

5. "The Business Case for Breastfeeding: Steps for creating a business friendly worksite," US Department of Health & Human Services Office on Women's Health, http://womenshealth.gov/breastfeeding/government-in-action/business-case-for-breastfeeding/employee's-guide-to-breastfeeding-and-working.pdf

Notes and Resources   233

Special Circumstances Appendix 2: When a Baby Dies

1. Child Health USA 2011, "Neonatal and Postneonatal Mortality," http://mchb.hrsa.gov/chusa11/hstat/hsi/pages/206npm.html.

2. Ibid.

3. "Stillbirth: Trying to Understand," http://americanpregnancy .org/pregnancy-loss/stillborn-trying-to-understand.

About the Author

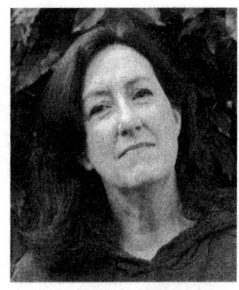

OLIVIA FAULKNER

Jeanne Faulkner is a writer, journalist, and registered nurse with over 25 years experience working in labor, delivery, and maternal-newborn health. She co-authored *The Complete Illustrated Birthing Companion* (Quayside Press, 2014) and writes the award-winning blog, "Ask the Labor Nurse," for *Fit Pregnancy* website. She's a senior writer and editor for the global maternal heath advocacy organization Every Mother Counts. She also blogs and answers readers' questions on pregnancy, childbirth, and parenting on her own website, JeanneFaulkner.com. She has written hundreds of articles, essays and op-eds for dozens of magazines on global health, maternal and women's health, human rights and poverty, feminism, politics, parenting, and more. She's the advocacy chairperson for the global humanitarian organization CARE's Oregon chapter. She lives in Portland, Oregon with her husband and family.

Acknowledgments

I count myself lucky to be surrounded by people who encourage me to go big or go home, to follow my heart and make stuff happen. First and foremost, I'd like to thank my husband, Jerome Faulkner, for his faith in me, his kindness and integrity, and for supporting me in a million big and little ways for more years than most of my readers have been alive. To my children, thanks for providing me with such a wealth of parenting experience and for making it easier for me to be a working mother than it is for many women. Only when you have children of your own will you understand how much I love you and how proud I am of each one of you.

My coworkers at Every Mother Counts inspire me every day to do my best work to improve conditions for mothers around the world. You're a motivating group of women and men who are smart as whips, funny as hell, and relentlessly high achievers. I'm proud to be included on this team and in your lives.

Thanks to my editors at Fit Pregnancy who allowed me to run my mouth off for eight years with my "Ask the Labor Nurse" blog. That's where this book started and I'm grateful to have been able to tell it like it is to readers who were hungry for accurate information, reassurance, and common sense as they navigated their pregnancies and births.

To Jenny Wapner and Kaitlin Ketchum, my editors at Ten Speed Press, thanks for believing in this book, for hearing me when I said, "it's for grown-up women, not children," and for supporting me to write a book that encourages women to approach their pregnancies, births, and healthcare as adults in charge of their own lives and decisions. Thanks to my copyeditor, Kristi Hein, for her exacting perspective and thoughtful questions that made this book that much better. Thanks to Chloe Rawlins and Emma Campion for designing a book that looks like it's for adults unlike so many pregnancy books, which look like they're written for babies.

Thank you to all the nurses, midwives, doctors, and most of all, mothers, who've taught me through your dedication, long hours on the job and in labor and delivery that pregnancy, birth and parenting are truly team efforts. When everyone works together, miracles happen.

Thanks too, to the team at Ten Speed Press and Penguin Random House for hearing me in that now is the time to change the way we talk about, think about, and approach pregnancy, birth, maternal health care, motherhood, and parenting. It is my hope that this book will help make that change.

Every Mother Counts

Every Mother Counts is a non-profit organization working to reduce the number of women who die due to complications during pregnancy and childbirth by raising awareness about the fact that even in the 21st century, these deaths still take place and up to 98% of them are preventable. EMC invests 100% of the funds raised through individual donations and product partnerships into programs that directly impact one of three critical barriers to maternal health around the world: lack of education, transportation and supplies. EMC is currently invested in 7 countries around the world.

Erin Thornton is Every Mother Counts' Executive Director. She joined forces with Founder Christy Turlington Burns to build EMC in 2010. She previously worked on the ground floor to build DATA and ONE as the Global Policy Director. She was a Presidential Management Fellow and worked at the U.S. Export-Import Bank as a country risk analyst for sub-Saharan Africa and at the U.S. State Department in the International Health Affairs office. She lives outside of Boston with her Husband and three daughters.

Christy Turlington Burns, founder of Every Mother Counts is a mother, social entrepreneur, model, and global maternal health advocate. She was named one of *Time's* 100 Most Influential People, *Glamour's Woman of The Year* and one of *Fast Company's* Most Creative Minds—all for her advocacy work to reduce maternal mortality around the world. In 2010, she directed the documentary *No Woman, No Cry*, which examines maternal health around the world and which inspired her to launch Every Mother Counts.

Index

Birth weight
    determining, 180
    neonatal mortality and, 225
Bleeding
    ectopic pregnancy and, 58
    implantation, 56
    during labor, 159, 160–61
    postpartum, 190, 198
    See also Spotting
Blood typing, 62
Bloody show, 111
Bottle feeding, 207–9, 216–17
Breastfeeding
    alcohol and, 214–15
    after birth, 181
    bottle feeding vs., 207–9, 216–17
    difficulties with, 209–12
    latch and, 211
    length of, 217–18
    pain management and, 189–90
    work and, 218–21
Breast milk
    donating, 215
    pumping, 212–13, 219–21
    storing, 213–14
Breathing, 131–32
Breech babies, 171–74

C
Cake batter, 41
Campylobacter, 41
Castor oil, 99
CBC (complete blood count), 62
Cervix
    dilated, 90–91, 114
    irritation of, 56
Cheese, 41
Chorionic villus sampling, 64–65
Cigarettes, 52–55
Coffee, 44–45
Compresses, hot and cold, 132
Constipation, 18–19, 158
Contraction and fetal heart
    monitoring, 70–71

Contractions
    pain and, 112–13
    Pitocin and, 148–50
    in prelabor, 112–13
    See also Labor
Contraction stress test, 71–72
Cookie dough, 41
C-sections
    baby size and, 85–86
    basic procedures of, 163–67
    for breech babies, 172, 174
    epidurals and, 146
    fear and, 163
    frequency of, 163, 169
    inductions and, 96, 97–98
    for multiple births, 172, 174
    newborn care after, 175
    recovery after, 167–68, 189
    vaginal birth after, 168–71
Cystic fibrosis, 63

D
Death, 225–28
Diabetes, gestational, 63, 64
Dilation, 90–91, 114
Doctors
    asking questions of, 65
    choosing, 27
    at delivery, 25–26
    first appointment with, 12–15
    inductions urged by, 85–86, 98,
        103–5
    types of, 26–27, 117–19
Doulas, 28, 29–31
Down syndrome, 68, 69
Drugs, 52–55
Due date
    calculating, 19–20, 66
    as estimate, 20, 103
    managing expectations around,
        102–3
    past, 20–22, 103–5

L

Labor
 bleeding during, 159, 160–61
 clothing for, 122–23
 determining start of, 107–14
 dilated cervix and, 90–91
 eating during, 125–26
 false, 112
 first vs. later, 127–29, 186
 hygiene and grooming for, 121–23
 lacerations during, 157–58
 leaking fluid and, 107–10
 old-school routines for, 123–25
 pain of, 83–84, 112, 129–30
 Pitocin and, 148–50
 pooping during, 159–60
 prodromal (prelabor), 112–14
 pushing during, 153–55
 stages of, 114
 starting naturally, 50, 98–101
 team, 35–38
 vomiting during, 159
 waiting for start of, 101–3
 See also Induction; Pain
  management
Laborists, 25–26, 118
Lacerations, 157–58, 189
Lamaze, 77, 131, 133
Latch, 211
Listeria, 41, 42
LMP (last menstrual period), 20

M

Massage, 134
Meats, 42
Meconium, 116, 151–53
Meditation, 133
Midwifery model of care, 6, 8, 29
Midwives
 choosing, 28–29
 first appointment with, 12–15
 in hospitals, 119

 transfer of care to OB from, 91–92
 types of, 27–28
Milk, 41, 44. *See also* Breast milk
Miscarriages, 13–14, 15, 17, 55–58
Morning sickness, 14, 46–47, 49
Motherhood, 223–24
Moxibustion, 172–73
Mucous plug, 110

N

Natural childbirth
 advantages of, 146–47
 medical intervention and, 78–79
 movement, 76
 See also Birth plans
Naturopaths, 26–27
Nausea, 14, 46–47, 49, 159
Neonatologists, 118
NICU (neonatal intensive care unit),
  181–83
Nipples
 inverted, 212
 painful, 209, 210–12
 stimulating, to start labor, 100
Nitrazine paper, 109
Nitrous oxide, 130–31, 135–36
Nonstress stress, 71
Nurses, 119–20, 176–77

O

Obstetricians, 27, 117–18. *See also*
  Doctors
Oligohydramnios, 87–88
Oxytocin, 145, 148, 190

P

Pain management
 approaches to, 130–31
 bathtubs, 132
 birthing balls and stools, 132

breastfeeding and, 189–90
breathing, 131–32
compresses, 132
epidurals, 29, 83–84, 126, 130, 136–47
hypnosis, 134
IV narcotics, 130, 135
massage, 134
meditation, 133
movement and positioning, 134
nitrous oxide, 130–31, 135–36
relaxation techniques, 133
Pap smears, 13–14, 63, 64
Parenting
challenge of, 222–24
fathers' role in, 204–6
reward of, 222
Partners. *See* Fathers/partners
Pediatricians, 118–19
Perinatologists, 118
Pitocin, 148–50
Placenta, functioning of, 103–4
Placental abruption, 87, 160–61
Polyhydramnios, 87
Postpartum period
depression, 188, 202–3
experience of, 185, 195–201
final checkup, 201
healing during, 188–92
sex and, 192, 201
Poultry, 42
Preeclampsia, 63, 64
Pregnancy
appearance and, 18–19
approaches to, 2, 6–8, 11–12
birth plans and, 79–81
eating during, 39–45
ectopic, 58
fear and, 2–3, 6–9, 94–95
finding out, 5–6
last weeks of, 93–105
length of, 20, 21
risk and, 7, 9–12
sex during, 49–52

telling others about, 16–18
weight gain during, 39–40
Prelabor, 112–14
Premature births, 21, 87, 88, 120, 181, 225
Prenatal education, 75–78
Prenatal tests
approach to, 61–62
diagnostic, 64–65
genetic, 64, 67–69
for moderate- to high-risk pregnancies, 70–73
routine, 62–63
screening, 64, 68–69
ultrasounds, 63, 65–67
See also individual tests
Prodromal labor, 112–14

Q

Quad screen, 64

R

Relaxation techniques, 133
Rh incompatibility, 10, 62
Risk factors, 9–12
Rubella, 62–63

S

Salads, 41
Salmonella, 41, 42
Seafood, 41, 42
Sex
postpartum, 192, 201
during pregnancy, 49–52
to start labor, 50, 101
Shaving, 123–24
Shellfish, 41
Shopping, 22–24
SIDS (Sudden Infant Death Syndrome), 225
Sleep, 47–48, 198–99, 201–4